I0437878

WILLING TO BE WILLING

God Can Work With Bad Choices And A Death Sentence

by

Johna Reeves Platero

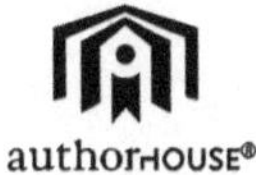

AuthorHouse™
1663 Liberty Drive, Suite 200
Bloomington, IN 47403
www.authorhouse.com
Phone: 1-800-839-8640

First published by AuthorHouse 6/25/2008

ISBN: 978-1-4343-2376-7 (sc)

Library of Congress Control Number: 2008900936

Printed in the United States of America
Bloomington, Indiana

This book is printed on acid-free paper.

Chapter One: The Meeting

Ken's point of view

The buzz around the camp was all about the new person and as soon as I entered the lunchroom I was hustled aside, "Did you see her?"

"Who?"

"Someone new," Brian whispered. "She's a lawyer."

"Hmmm."

"She's a redhead."

Brian was the local gossip. He hated that name preferring to be known as the information director among the small group of men I hung out with at this place we called the "fun world." He was 19, full of energy, himself and information. Brian was about 5'9", 170 pounds with black hair and French roast colored eyes. He was bright and funny and I liked him a lot. "Did you see her legs?" I had not. "Man," he sighed, "they're something." I was more interested now. "She doesn't shave them."

"Hmmm."

The food door opened and we pushed into the streaming herd. I hope I didn't noticeably gulp my food but I couldn't leave this room fast enough. And, I would have made a smooth exit too if it weren't for that Heimlich thing I suddenly needed. Just kidding! I burst from the cafeteria's double outer doors and snapped my head from side to side. I sought the redhead. I couldn't help myself. I started across the mostly empty courtyard toward the lounge when I spotted her. Now, less than a month ago I was pretty much doing what I wanted, when I wanted and how I wanted. At this point, I am serious about serving the Lord completely, but I can't say I was approaching this interesting woman to share my testimony. I stopped her on the sidewalk and introduced myself. Johna. I liked that name, Johna. I'd never heard it before. I made up some reasons to talk a bit longer with Johna and I was very impressed. She had beautiful eyes. She politely excused herself and left me standing there wondering.

That night partly because I couldn't sleep and partly because I knew my weakness I increased the fervency of my prayers. "God", I said, "You know me." I had been praying this prayer every day for nearly a month. "Help me wait on you, but I need a woman." Then I told Him what I wanted. That request varied but the gist of it was I wanted to fall in love with a woman who loved the Lord. It was my only hope for happiness.

Johna's point of view

When my sister and her family left me at the facility I knew that never again would I see them. I came to this place with a plan. The plan must be followed because it would end all the problems before me. I had no intentions of going to prison or even to be involved in a trial. So, the plan was simple. Go to a rehabilitation center, hide and take the medications that would end my life and would, if there were no in-depth investigation, look like I was ill with a blood disorder and/or was involved in an overdose of prescribed medication. Good luck on finding from whom or where the prescription originated. Though drug use or alcohol was not presenting problems in my life this would be the perfect place to carry out the plan. The place required attendance at one meeting a day plus the full campus afternoon session. Lunch was finishing and it was time to get to the required meeting. I scanned the campus wanting only to avoid all people. Not many were moving around as lunch was probably just finishing. There was the blond guy with the beautiful body. "Johna," I sternly told myself, "That is a beautiful piece of fluff and you need to stay away from him."

"Hello." It was Fluff and he had blue, really blue, eyes that seemed to look straight through me. "My name is Ken, welcome." We had a few more words but I knew that getting away from him was important. I hurried to the group session room wondering how to manage this place and the people so that my plan was not discovered or interrupted. I didn't want my Mother to have any more embarrassment or pain because of a trial where all kinds of facts about me would be disclosed. This needed to end.

In the group room the chairs were in a circle and a couple of people were already in the room as was the facilitator. I sat down. The room filled up and it seemed like the group was ready to start when the door opened and in walked the man with blue eyes. He sat across from me. I was glad that my white shorts and orange top were attractive and that I had a great tan that allowed the hair on the top of my thighs to glisten. He didn't seem to acknowledge me and I remembered that he must not become part of my plan.

The noise in the room was loud and I realized people were talking and there was a heated debate. I had zoned out of the group. Blue Eyes was talking really loud and I was impressed as he said, "The problem with you guys is that you think being happy is bad, that happiness is part of using so you all are upset because Darwin goes around smiling a lot. Leave him alone. Darwin be happy." Many of the guys clapped. The facilitator told Ken he was too simple and that he ought to work on his problems rather than hold on to the crutch he had built out of God. Hmmm. A man with a mind of his own. "But Johna," I reminded myself, "These are drug addicts and alcoholics. Don't listen to them."

Ken's point of view

It was early in the morning and I had been standing around in all the obvious places looking for her, but I didn't see Johna. She wasn't at breakfast or the early group session. At lunch I really was looking for her but she still was nowhere to be seen. I had the perfect approach. Darwin was to be honored for his birthday and we had a gift that needed wrapped. I would ask her to wrap it for us because everyone knows she would do a better job than a group of guys. On my way to afternoon group I literally ran into her. She agreed to wrap the gift following this group session. She had been placed in a different small group. I would see her at the laundry facility later. The group passed without one comment from me. The facilitator, Sue, commented that she was pleased I was listening and considering that I needed to do more work on my issues. She did not understand and it didn't seem she was open to hear why I was in drug rehabilitation. I thought about the group session the day before and what I considered the attack on Darwin. They called it being on the hot seat. I wondered what Johna thought about it. I thought the group was a joke. People sit around destroying one another, verbally and freely, knowing, I might add, that they are in the protected confines of the group where everyone is encouraged to talk. The hot seat technique put a person in the position of getting "feedback" and my day was coming. Darwin's experience could have been worse. I knew the claims and the premises about group therapy, but I didn't buy into the belief that this was the way to freedom from addiction. Most of the guys here had shared, privately, that they had tried this format previously and had stopped using, for a while. I thought about the people in the group and wondered again why I had been so sure that coming to this place was necessary. And on top of all this I missed my Dog Maddie. Maddie was a beautiful 70-pound female bull terrier and she loved me. She had been my companion in Wyoming and then back in my hometown of North Platte. She was at Dad's while I was in rehab and I missed her. In Wyoming she often went to work with me and stayed sleeping the whole 8-hour shift. And that dog, she could play soccer like a champion. She used a tennis ball kicking it with a front paw and one kick put the ball all the way down the hall. As soon as she kicked the ball she'd turn and guard the end of her hall. It was tough to beat her in a game of soccer.

In the group was Ann who was very quiet, white skinned with freckles and lots of blue eye makeup. She derived pleasure from cheating on her husband and, I think, more pleasure from talking about it. She was here to "get control of her drinking." There was Darwin who was a fat country guy who had to be in rehabilitation or his wife would leave him. He hated to talk about problems and basically wanted to be anywhere else with a bottle of anybody's whiskey. He said so. That true statement and his always-ready smile drove Gene, another group member, into a near psychotic rage. Gene, surely short for Eugene, was a 5'7" Karate black belt; over compensating macho man who was a little too convinced that he intimidated the entire world. Gene was in the throes of a two-year stint as a dry drunk. That means he has stopped drinking but still has the desire to drink and kept the behaviors of a drunk. Gene really hated the portly farmer, Darwin with his easy go lucky attitude. Darwin wasn't angry about being in rehab because he knew it was for 30 days. Thirty days and then he would be sober. Thirty days and his breathing would be easier, the tightness in his chest would subside, and his hands would stop shaking. Thirty days then Darwin would be home. Thirty days and he would have a drink. That kept him smiling. He'd already decided the dry and sober life was not for him but he would complete the program, make his wife happy and start over. As for Gene, well Gene was a believer in the system.

In the group where Johna saw and heard me I just had had enough. Gene told Darwin with venom you could smell, "You are fat and disgusting...nothing bothers you because you are too dumb to be bothered." Darwin looked up and there was fire in his eyes. He had heard all about Gene. Gene and his 3 time Kansas State Karate Champion, bone breaking reputation and strong believer in the rehabilitation model used by this center. Darwin smiled and then he laughed. Gene started a tirade against Darwin saying he wasn't man enough to keep his wife, and all eyes were on them, all eyes except mine. I was watching the newest member of our group. I had my eyes on the pretty, petite, redhead with fascinating eyes. I instantly knew two things about her. She had confidence and she clearly did not belong here. I could hardly take my eyes off her, but I was tired of listening to Gene.

"Why don't you shut up?" I said with some loudness of voice. The room went silent and our counselor sucked in her breath. "Gene everyone knows you don't know how to smile, but why do you care that Darwin does? Leave him alone." I don't think Gene was used to being addressed in that fashion. At first I thought he was going completely blue, he was so mad. Then I thought we might go at it, but Gene's wife pulled him back. They'd been to this rehabilitation center three times and she was hoping this time he just might find an easier way to be clean and sober. Sue made some comments and called for an adjournment and group was over. I caught the redhead looking at me but she quickly looked away. Gene, however, he was staring all over me. As I walked by him I said, "One thing about being here together, locked down so to speak, Gene you always know where to find somebody." Darwin stepped between us and I tried to see which way the redhead went. She was gone. "Let's go find Brian and the others," Darwin said. We chatted as we walked toward the recreation room, but I don't remember a thing we said. I was thinking about red hair and hazel eyes.

This story may read like fiction to some of you, like a fairy tale to others and some will think we just made things up to tell a good tale. In reality it is a love story, a powerful almost unbelievable love story that God allows us to experience. It is a story of natural love between a man and woman that is infused with God. God tapped Johna and me when we had nothing but shame to cling to, nothing to give of any value, no comforts and no privileges to lay down. We had made decisions that left us in chaos. We were not tricked, prodded, or deceived into wrong. We were sinful people who used and hurt others and ourselves. No one we cared about wanted to be close enough to us to help and we were not capable of helping ourselves. Our story would have been a tragedy of lost potential and ill used opportunity but for Jesus. We were two people who wasted life on selfish endeavors and schemes that never quite paid off. Without Jesus I can say with confidence that neither of us would be alive today. Enjoy this story knowing that in every life there is dirt, wrong, and ugly but Jesus has a way of using all that, if we are willing to be willing, and He will use it in beautiful eternally meaningful ways.

Johna's point of view

The noise from the campus awakened me. I felt shaky and strange. It had only been 2 or 3 days that I had taken the medication but I felt weird and paranoid. The noise was talking and laugher and the air conditioner running. The room was cold. I showered, changed clothing and stepped outside to see Ken, blue eyes, fly across the volleyball court and return the ball to score the winning point. Lots of yelling and clapping and suddenly Ken was next to me. "You look nice...what have you been doing?"

He was nice and it felt like everyone was watching us. I still am surprised at my return remark of, "I feel anxious." He said that he had the very thing to cheer me up and asked me to wait while he got it. He quickly returned bringing a cassette player with a tape already in it. "Listen to this," Blue Eyes briefly touched my arm. "It will help." I went to dinner that evening having listened to the tape. It was strange. A man was talking, reading from a book, and it was dramatized having the sounds of animals and other voices. I felt calmer. When Ken saw me enter the room he immediately left the dinner line and joined me at the end of the line. "What did you think of the tape?" He was so happy and attentive and when I asked what I had been listening to he looked astounded. "Johna it is the Bible from the book of John." Over dinner Ken talked and talked about this and that making me laugh. He would make gentle fun of himself and others and some of the other guys joined in with lots of laughter. Ken stimulated a sense of community and caused us all to believe that things would be okay. As we left the room he told me he'd be waiting near the ice tea station so we could sit together at the evening meeting. As I got ready for the evening meeting the tape finished playing and I started it again listening more closely. When I came to this place I brought two suitcases with me --all my possessions. Mother had given me, years earlier and in fact when I graduated with a Master's Social Work, a Bible. I opened it and cried. In a month or so I would be dead, the plan would have worked to save all of us from more embarrassment, but in that moment I was sad and missed my Mother and I wanted to be near Ken. I hurriedly dressed and went to the tea station. It was unreal to watch the people drink and drink and drink coffee and/or ice tea. When Ken approached me I commented on it and he told me that the caffeine helped with drug withdrawal and he encouraged me to note the amount of sugar each person put in their drink. The evening was a testimonial, Ken told me, given by a counselor named Tom. It was sad as he shared about his addiction and his losses and his relapses. Ken made comments of explanation and as we sat shoulder to shoulder. I felt safe. Maybe I told him that sitting with him left me feeling safe as a way to flirt but I really did feel safe when near him. He encouraged me to join the group later that evening in talk, volleyball play or board games. I left to my room.

Ken talks

I watched for Johna even while the guys and I talked. We always talked about God. The counselors were nervous about me and accused me of having a crutch saying that I was using God and religion to avoid dealing with the issues that had resulted in addiction. It didn't make sense to me that they were so against God and thought their way would really work when each of counselors had already shared about a relapse or two and the continued desire to use. It is true; in the two weeks I had been on campus I had found a niche of witnessing Jesus to the folks there in rehab. I now had four or five guys I really liked a lot. Besides Brian and Darwin there was John and Marvin, police officers with whom I immediately had rapport due to my former police officer status. And, there were a couple of black guys that I really liked, Robert who had used cocaine for years and needed a new way and there was Derrick a CPA who recently had fallen into cocaine use and could not find a way out. I was here having the rehabilitation experience paid by the Union Pacific Railroad where I had worked about 14 years and where my father worked and many other family members were employed. What was I doing in this place? How could this happen to a nice Christian boy from Nebraska? I was here by choice. Some of you have no concept of what a rehabilitation center is like and others of you cannot conceive of there being a need for such a place. If you took people from several parts of the country, and those were people who had depleted their hope, their health, their employers, spouse, and their families, then you would have a pretty good representation of the group at the center. Social misfits, the lot of the, but wait make that us, because I too was one of them. Even my family who completely endorsed my conversion could not quite get behind this rehab thing. I admit that I was quite nervous about this rehab experience. I never admitted to anyone that I had needs or shortcomings and now I'd be "sharing" with complete strangers. Remember I was Mr. Me and I didn't really care why everybody was here. I was here because God had convinced me that He was tired of my nonsense. I had been a lifelong yo-yo Christian. And at 34 I think God and I were both worn out.

The center or compound or campus as the rehab yard was called was really an old motel. You know the type, right besides a once bustling county highway and a few miles from the heart of a small town. The prospect of gain from the motel was lost many years ago and the owner had bailed happy to sell to the social service rehabilitation center.

In the summer of 1988 I completely left the way of my father. I come from a simple background and way of life. I was raised in a strict religious environment, my ethics and moral standards were high and I held what was to some an enviable position at my place of employment where I was paid better than average wages. My father, Harold, always loved me. I returned to North Platte following a difficult four years in Wyoming where working for the railroad resulted in always being cold. I came back to North Platte to be near family and to renew my relationship with God. However, I was quickly caught up in the lifestyle of drinking, dating, working all the possible hours and staying away from my dad and God. Years before I lost my daughters due to an ugly divorce and an inability to work out any kind of reasonable contact with them. I felt lost in the summer of 1988 and wished to die but knew and was afraid of the consequence of suicide. In July some friends and I became involved in shooting cocaine. In the course of a few weeks we used a lot of cocaine and I was offered the opportunity to move it on the rails and, in my position that would have been possible and would have brought a lot of money to me. One night three of us were shooting cocaine. As one person used the next became angry because he or she wanted a turn, now. I thought of the level of wrong in my life. In the middle of that evening we became angry and in the fight I hit and later learned had broken up the face of the other person pretty badly.
When I was alone, early in the morning hours, I cried out to God asking that He help me. I told Him that there was no way I could get out of the

drugs and the lifestyle that had consumed me. I told Him I would serve Him without compromise if He would rescue me.

About 10 a.m. on the morning that I had cried out to God the police arrived at my house, arrested me for assault toward the person I had hit and took me downtown. What

an experience. It had only been a few years earlier that I worked as a police officer in this same town. Many of the officers still had relationship with me. In one of my restless times at the railroad I quit and spent about a year on the police force only to return to the railroad where money and benefits made the job bearable. After being booked into the jail and given permission to shower, I bowed on my knees in that shower stall and thanked God for taking custody of me. I vowed to serve Him. I promised to no longer be an up and down Christian and I knew that God was tired of my games and this was the last chance for me with Him. In a few days I was released to expect further consequences at some later time. Within a couple of weeks following my release I checked with the employment assistance program and asked to enter a drug rehabilitation center. This didn't make sense to me or to my father who asked, "Did God deliver you?" I knew He had. There was no craving for cocaine or any drug, I was at peace in my heart and ready to deal with consequences and I knew that my face was like flint toward Jesus. And yet I also knew that I had to go to the rehabilitation center. It was embarrassing to me and to my father. All the railroad guys now had a label for me, drug addict. Yet, I had to go. I'll never forget my father's words to me, "I don't understand but I love you and I am with you. Do what you have to do." I couldn't explain to Dad but thought maybe I needed to go for humbling but no matter the reason I had to go. I really love my dad.

My great love for Dad became solid in August of many years ago, the year my 10-year-old sister Karla drowned. Dad often quoted the Bible saying "all things work together for good to him that loves the Lord." But, it was hard to see how Karla's death fit in this principle of truth. Karla's death was the beginning of obvious collapse in our home. Karla's death brought a sense of guilt among the rest of us. Instead of consolation and comfort there was blame and accusations. The atmosphere was charged with rage and then maybe a kind of resignation. And, out of that grew apathy. Mom left one day without a clue that Dad or I had noticed. Dad was devastated. He nearly lost his mind and I stayed with him as much as I could and talked with him from the Bible. I reminded him what the Bible said and though he didn't respond he continued to be faithful. He worked his eight-hour shifts and would come home and fall apart for some hours and sob himself to sleep. For years Dad was broken, and I didn't understand. I didn't know about stretching or testing of faith. I only thought about punishment and it wasn't that I thought my dad had committed some sin but rather that he was like Job being tested. It was scary. It was during this time that I started drinking. I was about 15 years old and had already tried pot. At first it was flavored vodka but I would get so sick and eventually I acquired a test for beer. Most of my friends were a couple of years older and getting something to drink was no problem. I stayed with friends who referred to me as "our other son" and I would see Dad every day but it was more and more difficult to witness his despair. I was gone all the time and though I didn't run the streets I was doing what I wanted and I was 15 years old.

The way I was raised to believe in God never left me but I put God on the back burner. I knew God wanted me but I became very good at just ignoring Him and doing my own thing. This rebellion has cost me countless hours of heartache. I was very selfish. If I wanted something I got it with little thought of the feelings or repercussions on others. You know, even now when I do something charitable it is often because of God's infinite grace and not because I have so changed to first consider another. A life of sin cannot be easily surrendered. It is like gaining an enormous amount of weight and the crash diet doesn't really help that much in the long haul. It takes time for old habits to disappear from our lives. That is why the Bible instructs us to crucify ourselves daily. I understand that habits and desires can be instantly broken by God's power and I have experienced that in the use and desire of cocaine, however, that is not what I'm talking about here. I am referring to those comfortable old secret sins that we've had for years. It may be a vice or a trait such as gossiping but whatever it or they are, we all have them. These things do not suddenly disappear but can be reduced as we yield more and more control to God's own Spirit. We must, as I told Johna long ago, be willing to be willing to have God more and more in our lives.

In those first couple of weeks at the rehabilitation center in Kansas I considered what an extremist I was. My bounces were like the super ball and usually public. And, there were many. Do you remember the toy super ball? It was smaller than a baseball and made of some space age rubber. It was so hard you couldn't squeeze it and really you could not even play catch with one. But there was something wonderful about the super ball that to this day is unmatched in balls. With the slightest effort you could bounce one higher than a house. Man those balls could bounce! For hours at a time we would throw one on the pavement and run to retrieve it only to throw it again attempting to loft it higher than the time before. There was no game associated with super ball and it came in one color and wasn't much to look at and its sole purpose was to bounce. The super ball provided mindless innocent activity that sold thousands if not millions of balls. For all the fun we had there was a flaw in the super ball. Sometimes they would break apart. Actually it was more of an explosion. The pieces of the ball would go in many directions. God help you if you were too close to the exploding ball. The thing about the explosion, you could not tell by the look or the feel of the ball that it was about to explode. There was no visible sign or indication of the impending letting go and destruction of the ball. My life I'm afraid was very much like the super ball. When I bounced it was high but sometimes the coming down was in many pieces often hurting not just me but whoever happened to be close to me. In all my life, until I surrendered control to Jesus, I did not consider myself a selfish person and that ought to have been a clue. The inconsistency of my character did bother me. I thought often of my Dad's faithfulness. He modeled what is right regardless of the cost and he served the Lord without waver even in the face of sorrow and tragedy. Dad never took a backward step and never turned aside from God's word and Spirit of Truth. I wondered what was wrong with me.

Knowing that I could describe my life as a super ball I felt, in this place of rehabilitation where the paradigm of treatment was not one I agreed, grateful. God expected a lot of me and I knew that though I was in a fix He would stand with me and it would work out right. Memories of Bible stories, portions of memorized scriptures, and sermons heard long before caused the fire in me to stir until there was an unquenchable need for God. He was all I could talk about and five of my buddies at the center prayed the prayer of salvation in the first two weeks of my stay. I knew what a godly man should look and smell and be like because of my Father's model. Though I had burned most bridges and was alone and unfulfilled and didn't believe in love because there was not one couple I wanted to emulate I knew my Father loved me. I knew Dad's love was real and that the promises of God to my Father were true and strong and that they applied even to me.

I smiled while waiting for Johna and thinking about my first inclination upon seeing this place. It was, run. Just floor this Ford and run. Actually on my arrival I hit the loose gravel on the pavement and the bald tires refused to grab when I braked. So, my arrival was noticed and embarrassing. The first meal can never be forgotten. I've never been a picky eater but 38 sets of eyes greeted me the first time I entered the dining room and some were hostile while others warm and kind. The ones I recall were watery and empty of comprehension or focus. The cooks were older women and friendly. That first day the food was creamed corn, creamed beets and meat of some type that too had been creamed. There was orange Jell-O salad with carrot shavings on the top. The food assortment was quite colorful and I found myself whistling Zip - a - dee - do -da.

There was Johna! I asked her to sit with me in the courtyard on a bench where flowers bloomed and the trees added to the coolness of the evening. Again I asked about the tape. She told me that she really didn't believe in God. There was nothing I could say. How could a person not believe in God? What was the matter with her? She conceded that she would not go so far as to call herself atheistic but she just didn't believe in God and called herself agnostic. That night we talked and talked. The stars were beautiful and the night was warm. I recall talking a lot about God and His love for me and how I knew Him but left Him and yet at my return He was there waiting ready to restore me. Johna was a good listener. When we left one another I took her hand and told her that I was praying for her. She smiled. I told her that it saddened me to see her taking her life and that I wished she would decide to live. She looked at me and paled and was upset as she left. As soon as Johna was gone I called my dad and told him that I had met a woman who did not believe in God and that if she left the center without finding Him she was going to die and go to hell. I asked him to pray and I told him her name, Johna. Once you are on my Dad's prayer list you will be prayed for every day for the rest of his or your life.

The next day Johna was at breakfast and she and I were together all day. Early in the afternoon I asked her to take a walk. We left walking toward the west and we walked and walked. After a while we held hands. Johna told me stuff. She told me stuff including why she was at the center. She was working to deal with an impending Grand Jury Indictment. I knew she talked to me a lot and had left many details out of the story, but I didn't ask. At one point on that walk we kissed and I knew the feelings I held for her were different. More than having her as a friend, a lover or a wife I wanted her to know God. I called out to God during the dinner hour skipping food to ask of Him for understanding and committing to not sin with this woman to whom I was so attracted.

In the next few days the center had recreational activities that included bowling, going to the lake where Johna and I walked which was 10 miles, and other group events. Johna came to all of them and she was always near me. On one of these days she asked if I was a FBI agent and on another she asked if I would leave the center with her going out of the states to a place where extradition would be difficult. In these exchanges I begin to see her differently and I prayed that God would let me see her as He saw Johna. I kept returning in our conversation about the position of her being agonistic. I confess I'd never heard that word. I was horrified. Funny, I had lived so close to the edge for many years, always pushing the threshold and yet now the thought terrified me. It seems that at last I had a sense of the loss the Christ in my life and would not allow Him to move out of center stage. I wanted Johna to know Him. In truth she scared me a little. She had seen things I had not even read about and she had a remarkable amount of education and social grace, but she didn't believe in God. That lack of belief in her kept me awake praying.

Johna talks

In the week after connecting to Ken I was near him all the time. When he was near I was not afraid, and fear was growing in me. He said one day, "Stop doing whatever you are doing that is going to kill you." I left him amazed wondering how he knew and that day I flushed the pills down the toilet. The only effect of that medication was weeks later when my toe nails all came off and I can only surmise the medication was the cause of lost nails. I didn't tell him that I stopped the medication because there were moments when I was sure he was the FBI spying on me and that any minute I would be taken away for some legal procedure. So, I decided that Ken needed a test and I would invite and compel him to have sex with me and then, he would probably have so much guilt, it would be easy to get him to leave the country with me. I would flee and hope extradition did not come my way. To my utter amazement Ken refused sex and steadfastly would not consider leaving the country. He did make an offer. He offered to marry me.

Ken's point of view

One day at the bowling alley I asked Johna to marry me. She laughed. I told her that unless she found God she would die and be in hell and I was not going to have sex

with her, live with her or leave the country with her but I would marry her and be her partner in whatever came her way. During the couple or three hours we were at the bowling hall I kept at Johna to marry me or at least go to the courthouse and get a marriage license. Somewhere in this we started laughing and to this day there has been no laughter equal to that day. I think it was the laughter that caused her to agree to get the license. The next day Johna and I left the grounds separately to meet at the courthouse where we applied for the marriage license. It was easy and we were full of laughter.

Late on the night we got the marriage license Johna and I were alone outside on the campus. By this time we both had been talked to by the administration. We were spending too much time together, there was too much talk about God and we were not working our programs. Johna had a difficult time being apart from me and I knew she had much fear about the upcoming legal proceedings that she believed would result in more embarrassment and prison. I hugged her and asked her, "Johna why don't you try God? You have tried everything else and nothing has worked. What do you have to lose? Just go to the chapel and tell God that you are willing to be willing to know Him." Johna returned my hug and kissed my cheek. She told me she'd think about it and left for her room. That night was another night of prayer for my new friend. In my time with God He gave me a great gift. He allowed me to see Johna like He saw her. Wow! I loved her more than I've ever loved another. I saw this woman whom God loved and for whom He had great plans. I knew that if she would find God she would be a person of great faith.

Johna talks

In the group sessions, every time, they first had each person say his or her name and then confess something like, "I am an alcoholic or drug addict." For some reason I could not play that game or state that lie. So for days I merely said my name and though the pause was awkward the next person would then speak. The counselor called me into her office and I told her that I was not an addict but had other problems. She merely shook her head and warned me that if I didn't work the program I would not graduate.

On the day Ken told me to try God I had been in-group and when there were no words of confession about my status one of the people in group very kindly asked what I felt about me. I said, "I am lost", and then I cried. There was a short pause by the people in my group and then the next person spoke. When Ken confronted me about trying God I felt like crying. Now, in my room alone I wished he would come to me. I hoped he would crawl into the window in the bathroom and then I laughed because that window was very small. I felt alone. At 2 a.m. I stood up, dressed and walked across the campus to the chapel. It was open and very small and pretty with stained glass art and a large window. No one was in the chapel so I sat in the front row. I carried my Bible with me and sat there for a while saying nothing but thinking about the mess of my life. A few months prior to this date I was teaching college, practicing some law and anticipating a new and wonderful career. Now there is only the impending disclosure of the wrongs in my life brought there by my greed and desires. I spoke out loud and simply, "God, if you are, please hear me. I declare that I am willing to be willing to know you. I need your help." I sat there a while and then went to bed and slept. The next day I told Ken and I told him that I had stopped taking the pills some days before. He asked me again to marry him. I told him that we ought to live together. He refused. I could not stay at the rehabilitation center. I was never an addict and the daily sessions were stressful and the counselors were very upset with me and asking questions about why I was there, what I was doing spending so much time with Ken and threatening to expel me and him. He was there paid by his employer and really needed, I thought, to complete the month. I told Ken that I was leaving. He offered the use of his truck asking me to return on Tuesday and marry him. I remember laughing. Many of the guys who were Ken's friends teased us a lot and there was a lot of laughter. Ken was serious and I knew that but thought if he finished the program we could leave and maybe stay together and I could not think about being separate from him because with him I felt safe.

I packed my stuff, checked out of the rehabilitation center and left toward my sister's house. Ken opened my Bible to Psalms and encouraged me to read as I drove because there was no radio or music in the truck and I had about 7 hours of farmland to drive through. As I made my way to Valerie's I kept reading, "Create in me a clean heart and renew a right spirit within me." I read and said it out loud over and over. It was late at night when I arrived at my sister's and an older brother and his family was there. We couldn't really talk until after midnight when my sister and her husband talked with me. My brother-in-law, Dale, asked what had happened to me. He thought I looked 100% better than when they left me at the center. And my sister told me I looked like death when they left me and that I really looked alive and well. So, I asked Valerie what she knew about the Man named Jesus. Valerie immediately cried telling me that for one year she and her children had, every night, prayed for me. She talked with me about her experience with God from the neighborhood church. It was a time of feeling close and I received forgiveness though I still didn't ask. The next morning Dale asked about the truck and I told them that I had met another man named Ken who told me about Jesus. I talked and talked about Ken telling them that he wanted us to get married. I laughed. They didn't and in fact Dale told me, "Go, marry him, I've never seen you appear so healthy." I called Ken and hearing his voice brought a quietness and calm in my spirit. In fact, I called him several times. Each time he encouraged me to come there on Tuesday before noon so we could get married. On Sunday afternoon I went to a church and picked up an old hymnbook. I took it with me reading the words of many songs.

Tuesday morning early I packed my stuff and left my sister's. I felt confused and conflicted. As I drove toward the center I sang the song that had stuck in my thoughts on Sunday afternoon, "years I spent in vanity and pride...knowing not my Lord was crucified, caring not it was for me he died at Calvary." I pulled onto the campus and was told that Ken had been asked to leave. One of the guys told me he was waiting for me at the courthouse and that I was late. I drove to the courthouse and Ken was waiting on the steps. He told me the Judge had a cancellation but she only had a few minutes before she had to leave. I reminded Ken that we didn't know one another, that legal matters were in my future and that I really didn't want to get married. He moved me along the steps into the courthouse telling me not to worry and that we'd talk about all those things after we saw the Judge. More than the conversation I recall the feeling of being safe and knowing that it would be okay. Robert and Derrick were the two guys who showed up for the marriage ceremony and they were our witnesses. We were married September 7, 1988.

That night we rented a motel room across from the rehab campus and invited the guys over to the room. We served them soda pop and chips. My aunt and younger sister sent a floral arrangement to the room. Ken's dad asked him, "What's going on?" Ken remained sure and confident telling everyone that we were supposed to be together and that everything would work out okay. The rehabilitation center had expelled him because he told them I was returning for our marriage and that I would stay the remaining three days of his program with him. They felt he had broken too many rules and would not allow him to graduate.

We were married. I'd look at him and smile. Ken so beautiful and he was so sure. The first morning I awakened to a cup of coffee and a roll and a fully dressed husband who read the Bible to me as I enjoyed the food. Then he prayed. My heart softened and I wondered just what experiences were ahead for us. We went to Valerie and Dale's. They were sweet and we stayed there a few days giving ourselves a chance to figure out just what we were going to do. I called my attorney and he expressed horror that I had married and told me to expect, within a couple weeks, being called by the Grand Jury. I promised to keep in daily contact with him. My youngest sister had a time-share in the Ozarks not far from Springfield where I would need to appear before the Grand Jury. She offered that we could stay there. So, Ken and I journeyed into Missouri and Arkansas seeing some of my family and arriving at the time-share. I'll never forget some of the comments that came toward us. My older brother was gracious but he warned us about getting too fanatically religious. My mother took Ken aside and asked him if he knew what he had gotten himself into. Ken told Mother that he knew and that things would work out okay and for her to worry no more. She shook her head knowing that we were doomed for more pain and yet another failed marriage. There were a few nights we stayed in various motels and it seemed like I had never slept better although Ken was tired and he was awake a lot. Sometimes I heard him praying. I felt safe. We arrived at the time-share to stay in a small camp trailer that was perfect. It was set out of the main traffic and no other people were staying in the area. It was in these days that I started calling Ken, Mr. Man. It seemed appropriate because he seemed bigger than life. I developed other names for him to include of course, Ken, but also Kenny, Kenneth, Vangie and Mr. Man. In truth, Ken has personality traits that fit all these names. It was fun being connected to him.

Ken's words

As we traveled toward the time-share we stayed a few nights in motels. It was one of the most powerful prayer times of my life to this date. I could not sleep but rather was awake praying. It felt like forces where very close and that Johna was going to be taken from me. One night we were in bed for some hours, Johna was sleeping soundly and I was drifting in and out of sleep when a loud banging knock came at the door. Johna was immediately in my arms very afraid. I called out asking, "Who are you and what do you want?" The response was, "I want my sister." I got up and put some pants on and walked to the door. Speaking through the closed door I replied, "Your sister is not here and in the name of Jesus leave." I opened the door and no one was standing there nor was any person in sight. That night I talked with Johna about what I believed was a spiritual war for her soul. We prayed or rather I prayed and Johna agreed with the prayer. When we arrived at the time-share I felt a restfulness and gladness in my spirit and we spent many happy days there waiting to hear from Johna's attorney that she had a date to come before the Grand Jury.

We immediately started reading, out loud, the Bible. Generally I read and Johna listened and asked questions. It was a fun exchange. I went through the prayer of salvation with her again so she would better understand what she had prayed at the rehabilitation center. I remember odd things about our honeymoon that still make me smile. One afternoon we skipped rocks on a lake in Arkansas, and one day we sat on a balcony terrace overlooking the streets of Eureka Springs, Arkansas. That day it rained and we were soaked to the bone, muddied and full of laughter. Those were happy days for us while we sort of put the world on pause and enjoyed one another. The night we went to the passion play was moving and beautiful. Several times I was brought to tears and saw Johna watching me. We built an altar to the Lord and made a list we burned asking Him to help us. Looking back I realize how odd I must have seemed to Johna, but I was so fresh from addiction I dared not dabble. It was all or nothing and I knew there were things I had to do that never before had I done. Besides, right away, God was answering our prayers. He began to build my faith and Johna's understanding and hope. We really were not thinking about any service we might ever do for God. We were trying to find out if we could face our own trials. Johna prayed I'm willing to know You God, but You are going to have to show Yourself. And so He did over and over and over. One night Johna cooked steak on an outdoor grill that is still the best I've ever eaten. We read Og Mandino, climbed a little, and we talked and talked. Johna was relentless about talking with me, and she expected me to talk back! I was amazed at all the topics she was privy to; her understanding and mind were fun to just witness. I'm not sure that even at night her mind stopped to rest.

It wasn't always fun and laughter in those days of discovery. We cried and fought back near panic a time or two. I remember the first of many nights we were together that I awakened praying in the Spirit and saying the name of Jesus. Satan wanted Johna to die and God snatched her from his grasp and Satan was mad. I know this because of the knocks at the door, a horrible oppressive gloom filling the space where we were staying and all the hair on my arms standing on end. Sometimes Johna would toss and turn and mumble incoherently but just as often she would blissfully sleep as I stood guard for her soul. Remember, God first showed me Johna through His eyes. I knew what she could be in Christ and you cannot stop loving someone when you see her as God sees her.

We called her attorney knowing that the days at the time-share were ending. He asked Johna who she knew that might be advocating a delay on her behalf. She laughed. There was no good reason why her case wasn't on the docket before the Grand Jury, but it was not. We fought against anxiety and doubt. Late in the evening we sat in a small boat on the lake near the time-share talking about God. I asked, "Johna, what would it take for you to really believe? A falling star?" Then I prayed for a falling star to bolster Johna's faith. We sat and waited. Later Johna told me she was formulating a response that would mitigate any disappointment I might feel when there was no falling star. At that moment it seemed the biggest star fell across the sky. We laughed and I started to pray when yet another star fell and I'm telling you it fell slowly from one end of the sky to the other. What a great conversation we had that night talking about believing in God and that in God all things are possible.

Johna's point of view

We had a few days left at the time-share and Ken was reading out loud from the Book of Job. I heard the words and thought on God. It then seemed as if I was stood on a balance beam and God was holding my hand. I knew that I could walk the beam with my hand in God's and life would be different and better than anything I had theretofore experienced. I also knew that I could let go of Ken and God would love and keep me, or I could really take hold of Ken's hand and there would then be more of everything. I paused as the realization of more love, more pain, more truth, more of everything settled on me. I knew in that moment that with Ken there would be some great sadness and I really thought about running or guarding my heart. However, in the deep of my spirit I pledged silently to keep hold of God's hand and to really and completely take hold of Ken's hand for better or worse. In many ways I gave myself to Ken that night on our honeymoon and it became and remains a milestone in my spiritual development.

Ken's words

There was to be no Grand Jury hearing so with the attorney's okay we left Arkansas and went to Nebraska to my dad's home. He was anxious and hoping the railroad would give me a break and allow me to resume my position. Dad talked with Johna a day or two and fell, I mean forever and ever, in love with her. The Spirit of God in Dad danced as Johna talked, questioned, reviewed and inquired about God. Every day for a month Dad hurried home from work to talk with Johna. We studied in the day and Johna knew how to study. Remember she was a recent law student and took the study of the Bible serious. We had great talks. She challenged Dad and me with her simple belief in God and His word. Even back then she confronted Dad about his lifestyle that denied any good pleasure like a wife in his life and queried him about his teachings and witness of Jesus. And she was my greatest advocate. She talked with Dad and me about why I would go back to the railroad where all I had experienced was making a decent amount of money and lots and lots of wrong decisions. She supported me in the decision that I must break away from the railroad. We loved her and prayed for her and entreated God to keep her from prison.

Johna talks

Ken's dad is really nice and his influence on Ken is strong. We were welcomed completely and the study of the Bible was fun. Ken's dog, Maddie, was another thing. I have never been much of a dog lover though I once had a cocker spaniel that was special. This dog, Maddie, was big and strong and different. Her vocabulary was impressive and she responded immediately to Ken's commands. For example, he'd tell her, "Don't watch us eat." Maddie would turn her face away from watching us and she didn't cheat by sneaking in a look or two. I was slow in developing a close relationship with this dog but came to love and trust her. In fact, later in Colorado it was Maddie that always helped me make it to the top of the mountain we regularly climbed. She also became my confidante listening to my thoughts and nuzzling me when tears flowed from my eyes.

Ken tells about it

After a few weeks I told Johna that we needed to go to Colorado. She called her attorney and he didn't care where she was as long as she kept a weekly contact with him. So, amid some parting sorrow with Dad, we packed the truck with all our belongings and left. I just knew that we needed time. I didn't know exactly where or how but we were on an adventure exploring how to hear and follow the leading of God. Within a few days we found the perfect place up the pass out of Colorado Springs. We rented the cabin that gave us a hot tub and a mountain to climb. We had very little money and didn't have jobs but we came day by day into the presence of God. I knew the word was the answer. His word is truth and life so we read it. We'd go up the mountain taking some cheese and bread and read for hours returning only when the coolness forced us inside. There was nowhere to go but to God for our needs. So, we went down the mountain to church and this was an exciting experience for Johna. She had never been in a Pentecostal church. I recall one of the first meetings. After the donuts and coffee for the early comers to church she asked, "What do we do now, work the crowd?" She made me laugh. A lesson about the body of Christ took on new meaning. One Sunday we left for church and I commented that perhaps we should return as the gas tank was near empty. We agreed that church was important and prayed. On the return trip back up the mountain the gauge fell way below empty and we had 22 miles up hill to get home. But the truck kept running until we pulled into the yard where it died completely out of gas. We celebrated God's goodness. One day we were eating what looked like black beans and tasted good to me. I asked about the food to learn Johna had used some decorative beans from a jar several years old. We would pray every day asking God to bring what we needed that day and to give us an opportunity in that day to speak His name. We ran out of money completely. There was no bank account or savings account or charge card or family from which to borrow money. We received money, a $20 or a $10, from unidentified people, from a last paycheck and from one or another family member just when we needed it. There was no need we had that wasn't provided during these months. It was the first time Johna had read the Bible completely through so we read it a second and a third time from October until April 1989.

Johna's thoughts

In these days of moving to and then living in Colorado Ken and I developed a saying, "What's the worst that can happen?" It helped us deal with the situation and caused us to keep trying to live by the principles in the Bible. Sometimes I goaded Ken telling him that the entire situation was ridiculous and that he ought not be surprised if I merely up and left because love wasn't really anything more than a trade-off. Ken generally gave a scripture back to me and/or took a walk only to return with a hug and an assurance that his love for me was beyond either of us. I knew that Ken had experienced problems with anger and believed that he would explode one day and that would be that, so I'd say things, little remarks about the past or a current desire for something more, trying to cause the explosion that would set me free. He had some anger but nothing that was explosive or out of line and that puzzled me. Much later he told me that he held onto the picture God gave him of me and was determined to stay in this journey with God.

Ken talks

One night our bull terrier, Maddie, was barking and acting crazy at the front door. I figured a house cat was in the garbage and opened the door only to let a brown bear sit down in the doorframe. Thank goodness the porch light momentarily blinded the bear and Maddie was quick in her nips and barking. I picked up the shovel and hit the bear on the head because I was afraid Maddie was going to be hurt. The bear wandered back up the mountain. What an experience. Maddie would growl at bears on TV for months after that event, but Johna and I, we smiled knowing that God was going to always bring adventure and excitement into our lives.

The mountain, about the second from Pike's Peak, was in our back yard and it was a five-hour hike up and back that mountain. I'm not sure how many times Johna and I made that climb but it was always special. The first time up we placed a pole with a flag with our names on it at the summit and each time there after we added a notch in the pole. There was something about being at the top of that mountain. In fact, Johna had encouraged me to finish a book, ELI, which I'd started years before and after being at the top of the mountain I could write it and finished it by the end of 1988. We talked about the writings and believed that someday God would use them to establish the GLORY FOUNDATION. We didn't have much of an idea what the Glory Foundation would be or provide but we really believed there would be a ministry that we'd get to be part of and it would serve last chance people like us.

Johna talks

Ken told me a story one day. I was amazed that he could so quickly tell the story but then it was over and the story was not complete. He laughed telling me it was a book he'd started years ago but had not finished. He called the book, ELI. I asked Ken about an outline or how the book ended and he flat out didn't know. He said the words came to him and that's how he wrote. I was enthralled and really encouraged him to write. The first five chapters he quickly wrote down as he'd written them long ago in his head. I went to the library to check the facts of these chapters. I had one legal size page of facts and every fact he had written was accurate. Life was amazing and exciting. Ken had a gift because he certainly did not have skill. He could not diagram a sentence and really wasn't sure about the difference in verbs, nouns or adverbs, but he could write. For a few months we lived Eli, Jasper and the other 13 characters in this book. A respect developed in my mind for Ken and I begin to see him as a person with unbelievable potential and I realized his potential would only be realized as he lived, completely, for God. The ending of Ken's book I realized opened the door to a sequel, which Ken needs to complete. It is called VISION. In those days in the mountains Ken wrote another book called GOD FRIEND. It is about the huge creature and his contact with man as well as his impact on the man.

In these days on the mountain I came to love Ken. When he prayed my heart and spirit was stilled and filled with hope and willingness. Late in October I told Ken one night after we were in bed that I needed something more. I explained to him that I believed that "God Is" and that more than anything I wanted to be pleasing to God, but I needed more of God in order to remain steadfast and faithful. Ken hugged me and talked with me about the Holy Spirit. Right away I loved the Holy Spirit, the teacher, the comforter and the helper. I wanted Him. Ken told me that in faith I could ask for the Holy Ghost to take up residence in my spirit and that He would, and Ken told me that often a person full of the Holy Spirit will pray in a new language, a heavenly language, that is by design made to encourage and bolster the person's spirit and faith. Yes, I told Ken, I want Him. So, Ken prayed and I wish you could hear that prayer. It sounded like music and as he prayed it seemed the room became full of this sweet and cool pink mist. Ken told me that God was among us and I know He was because things happened in my mind and spirit. I prayed to be filled with the Holy Ghost and rested in faith and love. It seemed to me that a memo pad filled the space of my mind and I saw four words written on that pad. I spoke the words and Ken prayed thanking God for filling me and giving me a new way to speak with Him. I was a little disappointed. Ken prayed so full and beautiful and there were four small words for me. Ken asked me to pray these words every day and I promised.

So, my habit became a morning time in front of the mirror in the bath room where I'd pray, "Today is the day You Oh God have given me and I will, yes I will, rejoice and be glad in it." And, then I'd say to God that really I didn't understand the prayer language but I wanted more of Him and I'd say the four words thanking God for the rescue He had brought into my life. By December Ken and I knew that we had to do something about the legal mess of my life. We called the attorney and in a few days he told me we could enter a plea that would release all the charges against me except the one of receiving stolen money and that was, in fact, what I was guilty of doing. So, some money came to us and I flew to Springfield staying only a couple of days to appear in court initiating the later plea. The days away from Ken were hard and I knew that without his influence I was weak and afraid. It was Christmas Eve when he picked me up at the Colorado Springs airport and we stayed quiet and alone during the holiday season.

In January 1989 we tried to find work but were not successful and God continued to meet our needs while we read the Bible and prayed hours every day. Ken called for us to have a time of fasting. So, for seven days we fasted and used the extra time to pray and read the Word. The fast reminded me of our honeymoon and the altar of thanksgiving that became a point of reference for us. One day Ken walked with me out into the Ozark woods. He had me gather a small portion of the foods we had and then together we wrote a list of things about which we needed God's help. There were ten items. Ken made a cross of pieces of wood and pine needles and he took some cedar wood and placed in on an altar he sit up with the stones from the area. It was a quiet moment for us. Ken then put the portion of food items and laid the original copy of the list of our needs on this altar. He prayed thanking God for His grace and goodness, for the plan He had for us and for the fact that He is the same yesterday, today and forever. Ken declared that we would trust in God and he started the fire. It burned. And then it started to rain. In September deep in the Ozarks it can rain and that day it rained. We were about two miles from the mobile home and we danced and shouted and sang thanking God for the cleansing of His Spirit that seemed so like the rain that soaked us until we literally had to wring out our clothing. Here is a note about the 10 items on the list. Every item God has answered except the publication of Ken's writings and this book is our first serious attempt to put his work on the market. God is faithful and He is good.

In April we moved to North Platte with Ken's Dad so we could be near the court as there were going to be hearings where I had to appear. These weeks of being with Harold were good for us. We painted his house and tried to cook and clean for him and every night we had hours of Bible study. And the end of May arrived and Ken took me back to Springfield, MO to enter the no contest plea. It was difficult. But, the year before May 1988, when I'd waived extradition and returned to my home town, and was placed in jail for several days until bail was posted, was much more difficult. The primary difference was that God and Ken were in my life and I was ready to deal with the consequences of my wrongdoing.

Ken's words

The month of June was painful. My hair turned white and we looked old and sad and we were. I thought God would work a way for Johna to be kept from prison. I could not see how such an experience would work good in her life or in our relationship. However, July 12, 1989 arrived and I took her to the federal prison camp near Phoenix, AZ. Johna's attorney was good at getting her into a new place where she would not have to sleep or use items that many others before her had already used. We were afraid and leaving her there broke my heart. I could not stay in Arizona because the charges on me for the assault had to be answered and my court date was scheduled for August 1989. On the trip from Nebraska to Arizona we listened to tapes, read the Bible and prayed. We were gentle with each other and I worked to assure her that though separated by prison we were one in spirit and God would work good in this for us. Sometimes it seemed like empty words but we refused to allow anxiety or fear to enter our minds and hearts. One of the tapes had a healing message on it. As we listened to the tape we heard of a healing to a neck and back. Tears ran down Johna's face as she told me that she could feel the heat in her back and neck and all the pain she'd been experiencing was gone. As we neared the prison we prayed and I told Johna that I believed she had two special angels assigned her. One was named Zebulon meaning constant and the other Sheka meaning instant. I encouraged her to know that God is constantly and instantly with His people to protect and to work His good will in them. We kissed good-bye.

Johna's point of view

The federal prison camp was clean. I waited in a lobby after Ken left me at the door. I was to see the administrator of the camp. She was very clear and direct with me. She told me that it didn't matter that I had a law degree nor that I had practiced social work or facilitated group therapy. I was in prison and if she learned of any legal or social work practice she would immediately have me shipped out of her yard. She explained that would mean I would go to Lexington, Kentucky and the route would include staying in jails across the states and the shipment would include both men and women. She asked if I understood her and required me to repeat her warning back to her. I left the office feeling numb and marked. The first step on the prison yard is forever imprinted on my mind. It was hot, the sun was very bright, and some women were raking the yard, which was dirt. The buildings were placed in a circle with the center area vacant except for concrete sidewalks. I later learned the track was behind the cellblocks. I recall standing there saying, "Oh God You are here and I ask that Your Holy Spirit walk before and behind me protecting all I do or say." I thought of the angel assigned to me and called on them to be my front and rear guard. This became a constant habit and I never left the cell without pausing to request the guarding from the angels and the Holy Ghost.

A guard instructed me to pick up the prison-approved belongings. As the guards went through the things I had brought, and they were those listed as okay by my attorney, I heard over and over, "Not this." Eventually I was allowed to take 5 books, three pictures, a few ink pens and tablets as well as the stamps and my Bible. The rest of the belongings I could send home if there was money in my account or if I wanted to mail them COD or they could be thrown away. I elected to throw the stuff away having no money and realizing that the stuff was not really that precious. The laundry was an interesting stop. The woman who ran it became a friend, Marcy. She was a young black woman from Missouri who was friendly to everyone. She gave me new items and when the guard left me in the laundry for a few minutes she encouraged me to do my own laundry paying the 50 cents per load rather than have it done by the prison where I would not get the clothes assigned me returned. It was good advise. Marcy, months later, had me speak with her grandmother on the telephone. She wanted me to testify to her grandmother that Marcy was "off the fence".

In other words, Marcy came be a place of serving God with her whole mind and spirit. We attended the Prison Fellowship meetings and prayed together every day, but what really impacted Marcy was that she started reading her Bible and her family at home prayed for her. Her grandmother had called the family together and gave an instruction the day after Mary was incarcerated. Each day for 40 days the family gathered 5 p.m. and ate together, the only allowable meal of the day, and then as a family they prayed for Marcy. Furthermore they were too pray for her all day long. Grandmother promised me that she would add my name to her prayer list. I would have loved to know Marcy after prison. She was one of the few African American women who did not get a sentence reduction. Marcy was from Popular Bluff and if anyone that reads this story knows her I would really like to talk her. It was against the rules have contact with another ex-convict while on probation. I followed the rules carefully.

The guard walked me to the cell block, showed me a two bed cell where I would have a roommate and then assigned me to the work detail of raking the dirt yard five hours a day. It was lunchtime and he told me to stay in the cell until after count. So prison was the start of the second phase of the life of Ken and Johna Reeves.

Chapter Two: Prison Days

Johna's point of view

Ken and I may write a book just about these 14 months and particularly about the exchanges in our letters, but a statement about these days is necessary for you to know how we were formed, during that experience, for today. I felt nothing the first weeks of being in prison and day by day kept my mouth shut, my eyes open, and my mind on God knowing that His promise is to work together all things for those who know and serve Him and that He allows nothing too great for His person to bear. I knew there was no defense and nothing that could be done for my release. Within two or three days of being in prison the letters started arriving. In another book we'll share some of those letters with you; however, you must know that every day I was in prison a letter from Ken arrived. I was the only person on that yard that received a letter every day and the women eventually asked about the faithfulness of Ken's writings. It was from that inquiry that I first read ELI to a group of maybe 20 women and then a second time to a group of 60 women. It was fun hearing them pick a character, cheer for that character and eagerly ask when the next reading could happen. THE PARABLE OF THE FRUIT, a small book that is published was a letter Ken wrote me during the last months of my incarceration. Some days I was the only woman in my cellblock that received a letter. My Mother was also faithful to write to me and I faithfully wrote her at least once a month because I knew it was part of the reconciliation process and I missed her so much. Toward the end of the months in prison I wrote Mother a letter simply telling her that I had been wrong, that I had lied to her and that her forgiveness was important to me. She forgave me.

There was no reason for me to be in prison. I had a great family and was brought up with values, education and care. There is no horrific event or trauma that can explain the why of my law breaking activity. I was arrogant and greedy and took where and what I could. My Mother, Helen, was in my opinion the best. She was always interested in what we were doing and enjoyed our schoolwork and good marks. She was the best encourager I've ever known and I always thought she loved me a little more than her other children. I'm pretty sure my siblings would disagree because when you had her attention you were all she cared about. The grief I've experienced because of the pain I brought her changed me. Mother visited me only a month before her death in December 2000 and encouraged me to "follow what God has put in your heart". Sometimes I still pick up the telephone to give her a call. There was never a call between us that failed to encourage me. I miss her. My Mother told me that though her mother had been dead 20 years she never stopped missing her. I now understand. Mother had this funny habit. She'd say, "Come children." It was always a surprise to me what that "come" meant. I recall one day it was pulling weeds in the garden and another time it was my favorite blackberries over homemade biscuits and yet another time we walked to the back of the property just for fun. I wish for all children this kind of mothering experience.

Ken's point of view

Johna was in prison and I was stuck in Nebraska. Remember the assault charge against me due to hitting the person with whom I smoked cocaine. Well, it didn't just go away and I was sentenced 90 days in jail expected to serve 72 and then have a time of probation while paying restitution. The color of the cell was green. Not grass green, lighter. Not mint green, but darker, dirtier, chipped and scarred. I lay on an iron bunk of the same dirty shade of green. A bed 75" by 30" in a cell of just 7 foot by 9 foot left little room for the four prisoners assigned to each cell. The two "bunks", a common sink and toilet made up the room. Actually the toilet and sink was one unit dented and battered from countless frustrated attacks. There were four cell rooms connected during limited hours of the day by a narrow four-foot walkway or hall. A single shower was on the south end of this walkway. This particular unit was called Federal. On the bottom bunk, face up and hands behind my head to provide a pillow, I stared at the bottom of the upper bunk. In pencil someone had sketched an elaborate portrait of the Virgin Mary. Funny I thought how being in jail makes you think of God. I had been trained to think of God. Every time the church doors were open we where there. I had thought of God as a demanding taskmaster incapable of tolerance for anything but total obedience. God was strict, harsh and unrelenting. If you didn't fear Him it was because you didn't know Him. There are a lot of lost people in jails. This wasn't the case with me. I was in jail because I'd been found. In being found I had found love and it grieved me that Johna was too far away and much too alone. I could do nothing but what I could do and that was to pray constantly for her, read the Bible and write her every day. I could and would do that. God gave me some good writings for Johna and I love the book we've put together about the prison days because it contains some of those lessons. She was faithful and wrote a daily letter to me. This exchange was precious. After about 45 days in jail I was allowed work release and it was good to have phone calls with Johna, work to earn money to go to Arizona and to spend time with Dad. He always fixed dinner for himself and me and we prayed for Johna. There was sadness in those days that I still can't explain. I really missed being with Johna, and I hated the fact that I could do nothing to comfort or protect her. God reminded me that the most important thing I ever did for Johna was to pray.

Johna talks

In the months of July through August I became like a piece of furniture. No one noticed or asked anything of the old chair that merely sat in the corner. Days would pass with not one word coming out of my mouth. I changed. My daily routine included the raking in the yard, 3 or 4 hours on the track where I learned to pray and another 3 or 4 hours reading the Bible. Nights were noisy in the cellblock with women calling out, laughing, swearing and sometimes crying. Sleep came in quick short spurts. The time on the track became very sweet for me. I recall asking God for a daily appointment. The track opened at 6 a.m. and I was already ready and generally the first on the track. God always was waiting for me and it wasn't long into those appointments that I brought up to Him my lack of knowing how to pray. Ken did most of the praying in our life. I did not know how to pray but as I read the Bible the Holy Spirit impressed on me to pray the Bible. The first prayer was out of Ephesians where I prayed that God would give Ken, my husband, a spirit of understanding and wisdom so he could know the hope to which God called him. I was praying the Bible that brought great change to my way of thinking. I recall when the Spirit of God, through Ken's writings, convicted me at a deeper level of my sins. I had prayed the prayer of repentance but until that day on the track I really had not felt the enormity of sin in my life and the hurtfulness of my actions toward others and especially toward my family. Of course I wanted to write each of them asking forgiveness and giving a kind of defense in that I was a changed person. God is so smart and I read in the Bible about God being our defense and how if we try to defend ourselves He won't. Well, I knew there was no defense for my actions and the only hope of any peace and reconciliation would come as God worked in me. So, I kept my mouth shut. My Mother wrote me, her sister wrote to me and my two younger sisters wrote me. Valerie and her family visited me in prison as well as Harold, Ken's dad, and our friends the Wilkes from Nebraska. However, the exchanges were surface and careful. However the reconciliation with my family came over the following years in various methods and disclosures.

In October Ken came to Arizona. The first visit in prison hurt so much I was physically ill following it, and I think Ken was not only ill but also uncomfortable. He arrived in Arizona in a small car my brother-in-law, Dale, gave him and he had to sleep in it because of Maddie and the lack of money for a motel and food. It was good to see Ken. He was beautiful and he brought the peace of God with him. It became a habit that he was the first on Saturday mornings for visit. And, by the time he was in the visit room some woman had informed me, "Ken's here and wearing his blue pants and that nice white shirt. He looks good today. Tell him hi and we want more stories." Marcy would braid my freshly washed hair on Thursday night. She'd braid it in cornrows and on Saturday morning it looked as if I'd had a perm. We called it the prison perm. My hair was very gray and had grown past my shoulders. Some of the women gave me skittles telling me to melt them and use the color for eye shadow. I passed on that prison beauty tip but I did use the desert plant root to bring some color in my lips. Ken was never late.

It was about this time of my days in prison that two events caused me to thank God for His presence. Often when I walked the track, and by now I was walking 4 to 5 hours a day plus running 3 to 4 miles four times a week, it was hot. One day while praying I realized it suddenly was cool. A cloud covered the sun. As the days grew cooler I had only a sweatshirt and one day Marcy, my friend who managed the laundry, brought a newly arrived brown prison jacket to me. This was special because there were not enough for everyone. The second awareness was that my New Balance tennis shoes that were very much worn out at the time of my arrival in prison were holding up to all the walking and running. In fact, they seemed in better shape than when I first came into the prison. It is the truth that those shoes served me all the days of prison. This is huge because the prison issued steel toed shoes were awful and caused problems with my feet. I had to wear them to work but could not have spend hours on the track walking in them. About a week after my release from the prison those tennis shoes simply fell apart. I mean the sides came away from the soles and the shoe was no more. But, in the days of prison they were great.

By late November Ken had the respect of the guards and they allowed him to bring the new manuscript he was writing into the visit room. It was wonderful to read his writings. This book took about two months to write and is called THE VIAL SO PRECIOUS. It is a great story about Agar, a Jew who did not believe in Jesus but knew that some did and that he would be able to sell a vial of the blood of Jesus if he stole it as Jesus died. The story unfolds as the blood of Jesus impacts Agar. I love this book and enjoyed reading it during part of our visit times. You know, Ken really suffered in those months. He could not get a job, he had little money, was often hungry and cold due to a lack of utilities, he knew no one and yet he came into prison full of the Holy Ghost and the knowledge that God is good. He was contagious.

Once we had a table but agreed to give space to another woman and her visitor. However, as they took God's name in vain and talked ugly and negative Ken gently told them, "It is not okay for you to sit here and take my Father's name in vain." They apologized and changed the nature of their conversation to more uplifting topics. If you can't say something lovely and good and lift up Jesus just be quiet!

In November the administrator called me to her office. She told me that she was concerned about a woman who could not get an immigration hearing while in prison and she wanted me to work on it. She agreed to give me written permission and to allow me to review the sentencing reports on any African American prisoners that wanted me to review their paperwork. This was in the day when the new federal sentencing guidelines had been instituted in an effort to make the white collar criminal serve time equivalent to the drug trafficker and it was based on the value of the crime. This changed the dynamics of prison life for me. I had permission to do some legal work. The Hispanic woman never got her immigration hearing during her time in prison; however, she and I became friends. She was about 35 years old and was in prison because her husband asked her to take a package to a friend across town. They lived in California and the person she delivered the package to was a FBI undercover agent and the package was a kilo of heroin. She was offered a plea but refused to testify against her husband. So, she was sentenced to five years and left four children at home and the youngest was six months old. One day she received a large envelope in the mail. The number of women getting mail was small enough that it was easy to notice her envelope. Some time later I was passing through the hall on my way to my cell and heard her crying. She told me that she could not open the envelope and then she showed me a stack of maybe 30 envelopes all unopened but one. The first envelope she received contained pictures of and drawings by her children. She had been in prison over 3 years and had not seen her family during the entire time. She could not handle the pain of seeing her children's faces. Several days later I asked her about praying and she talked with me about saying the rosary. I encouraged her to say a new rosary, one that contained the name of Jesus and asked that He give her strength to open the envelopes and to respond with courage and in the best interests of her children. Some days later she came to me with many smiles and asked me to come back to her cell. She had opened all the envelopes and had stacks of pictures for each of her children. She also told me that she now knew Jesus differently, and all her prayers where in His name. A couple years after prison I learned that she returned to her husband, forgave him and together they and their children are living a Christian life.

The black women were a source of joy and work for me. During the months I was there many of them had me complete the form asking for a reduction in their sentencing and most of the ones that filed for the reduction were awarded some less time. The most dramatic was an older black woman sentenced 10 years and had served one when we completed the request for a reduction in sentencing. She received a reduction of five years. She went from looking at another 9 years to expecting only 4 more years in prison. The black women honored me and would sing the ole' spirituals night after night during the hour or so we could sit in front of the cellblock. I've never heard better singing.

By this time the prison was pretty full, about 200 women, and I was moved into a cell by myself. No one else wanted the cell because it was directly across from the guard station so there was a good bit of noise during the night. The privacy was a good trade off for me. In the cellblock where I lived there were about 50 to 60 women with 25-30 on each floor and each floor had a room of showers and toilets. The cells had three walls to the ceiling but the front wall was merely eye level so the guards could walk by and see into the cell and there were no doors on the cells. There were advantages and disadvantages to this system.

In early November the administrator called me into her office again and told me I was being assigned a new work detail and that doing a good job could earn me a five-day furlough from the prison in about February. The work assignment was the lobby of the men's medium secure facility, which was located about 1/2 mile from the women's camp. She told me that this was difficult work and that a problem had been the attempted contact between women assigned this position and the men in the prison. She expected that would not be a problem for me, but told me there would be no helper for me in this job. It was difficult. The daily routine included cleaning large windows that required a ladder, cleaning the guard's restroom, mopping and buffing the large tile floor area and cleaning the floor and windows in the locked pass space between the lobby and the yard of the men's prison. Then about every other week a load of men prisoners were brought into the prison and the chains caused the wax on the floor to be scuffed so I had to buff using a different pad on the machine, give a thin coat of wax and then buff again. On those days I would work early in the morning and again during most of the afternoon. The other days I could do all the jobs by working two hours in the morning and about two hours in the afternoon.

My usual daily routine changed with this new job to include a work time from 6 to 8 or 9 a.m.; on the track until lunch when I would get uncooked vegetables and perhaps an apple and return to the track until about 1:30 and then until 3:00 to work in the lobby. At 3 p.m. I showered and put on clean clothing and was ready for the daily count that required everyone to be in her cell standing at the door at 4 p.m. Following that count was the mail call with dinner at 5 p.m. and then I'd walk the track for an hour or two and spend the rest of the evening in my cell reading the Bible. There was another evening cell count but I can't recall what time that count happened, but I know at 4 a.m. there was a cell count that was noisy and the guards used a flashlight to check on the inmates. It was my custom to get up and dressed before the guards entered the cellblock to complete that count. There was no rule about the TV going off or people going to bed though everyone was encouraged to be and remain in their cell after midnight. The floor where I lived was good about privacy and having lights off by midnight. Other counts of the inmates were called Census Counts and could happen whenever. At those counts you were to be at whatever job you were assigned. So, if it was 11 a.m. and Census Count was called and I was on the track I had to return to the lobby of the men's prison to be counted. These counts could take an hour or longer.

Everywhere I went on the compound I took my Bible. It caused me to feel safe and I could spend the time reading. Other than reading the Bible I read 4 or 5 books that Ken recommended but did not waste my time on junk reading. During the time of being incarcerated I watched one movie. Partly the TV and VCR were items about which the inmates fought and I kept myself out of all situations of conflict. I was in good physical condition from all the exercising but had to pay attention to eating. The inmates were very centered on food and were often rude and pushy during the meal times.

One day I was walking the track praying when a special exchange occurred. You know the prayer language of four words had continued to be just that, four words. I would pray the Bible and from time to time speak these words. Walking the track was a place of privacy. I walked alone most of the time and prayed out loud. No one cared or paid much attention. A friend, one of three people I consider friends from this time, walked past me and said, "Johna, God has dominion over me." I asked her what she said and she told me that she was merely telling me what I was saying. She had studied languages and I was speaking a Latin/ Spanish mix that translated to: "God has dominion over me." I thanked her but let me tell you I ran to my cell and wrote a letter to Ken. For more than one year I had every day, at least once or twice, taken time to declare that *God has dominion over me.* From that day on my confidence in God was strengthened and I was more resolved and willing to know Him in the deep parts of myself. The prayer language changed after this to include a very guttural sound and as I prayed it seemed like the taste and smell of dirt was in my mouth. I think this was part of the development of spiritual senses. To me the best part of this experience came the day when I smelled myself as clean. I'll never forget that day when I knew that I knew that God really is and that His love for me forgave everything. When I looked at myself in the aluminum mirror I was okay and could see some of mother in me and I thanked God for rescuing me.

The woman who gave me the translation of the prayer language was very special to me. She was the only other woman on the compound with a college education and she was kind and sensitive toward me. Her mother became a friend to Ken and for that I always have a place for them in my prayers and regard.

God is faithful and following my understanding of what I was praying He began to show me the wrong, the sin and the hurtfulness of my past life. It was weeks of walking and praying in repentance. God would show me behaviors or thought constructs and I'd realize the wrong of them. My heart was broken. It seemed like all that I thought and did was being bulldozed and the more time spent with God the more excited I became about the process. After some weeks of this work Ken's letters begin to speak to me about the grace and love of God and I recall the day when I again accepted His forgiveness. I understood that many people might never be able to forgive me and that there were relationships I had valued that might never be repaired, but God loved and forgave me. In that day the bulldozer seemed to push all the past, all the ways of reasoning and planning, all the hopes and plans I'd held away from me. I was free. There is no way for me to really tell you how I felt. It was one of two or three times I cried while in prison. They were tears of joy and relief. You see I came to know that GOD IS and because He is there is a system greater than me. That also means there is a plan for me that is greater than anything I had theretofore considered.

This book isn't about all the events of prison, but I must share how my prayer life changed. I would read the Bible and that is all I could pray. There was no agenda except His and there was nowhere for me to learn of His agenda except in the Word. In those days I'd write some scripture on 3 x 5 cards and pray it as I walked the track. Some of my favorite and most of what I prayed was for Ken. It was interesting to me that there was no time of praying for myself. God taught me a couple things through this process of teaching me to pray. First, in the position of wife I had and have a first obligation and that is to pray for my husband and, this is so cool, as I pray for him I really am praying for myself because we are one. Secondly, if I live in obedience to His word there is no reason to spend hours praying for myself. He is faithful to do the good work He has started and He will work everything for good to those who love and serve Him. I continue to have relief from this learning. From Revelation, you know it says in that book that if we read it out loud in the assembly we will be blessed, I prayed that Ken would be rapt in the Spirit and that he would have a voice to the church. The Holy Spirit opened my eyes about the church and filled me with love for His church. Ken was having some of the same understanding and it is no surprise that part of the mission of Casa Gloriosa is to encourage and strengthen the Church. By the way, I read the book of Revelation out loud several times while in prison. I was blessed over and over.

Ken's words

I left Johna after our first visit in prison feeling drained and yet resolved. God had not only kept her but He had built her faith. She was no longer dependent on my belief and faith, she knew God for herself. She looked more like the person God showed me when I saw her through His eyes. Now what? I have a little money, a car full of all the possessions we had, a dog and no idea where to go. There was a person in Tucson who had offered to help find an inexpensive place to live and thought there was a job waiting for me. So, I drove to Tucson after the visit and rented a cheap motel room. Maddie and I were exhausted. The next day the person had neither a place to rent nor a job, but I liked Tucson and started looking for a place to rent. That night I felt really discouraged as Maddie and I spent some money to stay in yet another cheap motel room. Johna would get a furlough in February if I could get a place with a telephone that could be checked out by the probation officer in early January. I had to find a place.

The next day I looked the house over from the west sidewalk before entering the chain link fence gate. I liked it. The house was white stucco freshly painted. You stepped up one step to the porch that was encased in six-inch square posts. It would be a real nice place to sit and watch the sun sets that this part of the world is famous for, but the more I looked at the place the more I doubted it was affordable. Too bad, Maddie would have loved the large fenced yard. I saw someone inside so I knocked softly and waited. A rather large man opened the door. He had rugged features and was a little more tanned than his doctor most likely would have preferred. He smiled and said, "Damn paint, it makes you goofy, name's Danny, what can I do for you?

"My name is Ken Reeves, I was told you have a house for rent?"

"Yes, I might someday. This place is taking more fixing up than I figured. It ought to be ready in a couple of months if I quit finding new problems"

"Well thanks for your time but I'm afraid I need something right now," I turned to step off the porch and asked, "What will it rent for when it's ready?"

"I don't know I reckon $475 isn't out of line."

"Thanks Danny," I said turning to leave. I crossed the street and heard him calling out to me.

"Hey! Hey Kid." I knew he was yelling at me and that he must need glasses. At 35 years I had longed stopped being a kid. He waved to me to come back and, like a good kid, I did. "Listen Ken, I was thinking that if you wanted to use the part of the house I'm finished with, and you don't object to my coming and going and working on the place, well it might work out. How would $200 a month be? And, you can move in tomorrow."

I said a silent thanks to the Lord and told Danny that would be great. He really liked Maddie and the utilities were already on so all I needed to do was get a phone connected. Most of the work still to be done on the house was outside and the place was really great. I stood amazed at God's direction and love. Danny could not possibly know how desperate for a place I was or that Johna could only come to me on furlough if I was settled. The probation officer could come right away. And, as if that were not enough I was keenly aware that the full amount of my worldly goods would let me pay the $200 and that would be just all I could pay. I didn't know how the phone would be connected or what would pay for the dog food, but I knew the Word and experience that taught me that tomorrow will have worries and anxieties of its own and that He had taken care of the need of today.

After moving into the house I started job hunting. I have always had a job. At 12 years of age I washed windows and from then on worked. I hired on the railroad at age 17 and was a foreman at age 21. I know how and have always worked so I started looking for employment having no doubt that I'd be with a job in a day or two. In the first two weeks I completed 33 applications and they ranged from mechanic to cook at a fast food place. No one would hire me and in the mail came some money that the railroad had not paid so I paid for a phone to be installed, set aside rent money and planned the rest for gas to see Johna every Saturday morning at 8 a.m. And, I started writing. I wrote two months on THE VIAL SO PRECIOUS. I lived John's grief as Jesus died and Peter self-loathing at the betrayal of Jesus and I changed. My love for Jesus became intense and renewed and strong. I realized all He did and gave and He did it just for me. I took the manuscript into the prison and the guard allowed Johna and me to read it. It was fun to watch this one guard stand close to the table where we sat so he could hear the reading of the book. When it was finished he told me it was a "good job".

The Monday after reading the last chapter of the VIAL SO PRECIOUS I was impressed in my spirit that I must walk carrying a sign that read LET ME TELL YOU ABOUT JESUS. I really did not want to do this but knew it was necessary. If you know Tucson you will appreciate that I walked from Alvernon to Oracle along Speedway and then back along Ft. Lowell. I was out that day about 12 hours. At different points I stood at intersection and watched the drivers. When they saw the sign they would quickly look away, smile, frown or sometimes shake their head. At one intersection I counted more than 120 cars in one hour so I was encouraged that many people saw the name of Jesus lifted up on that day. I was tired when I reached home but knew God was pleased with me. The very next day I was called to work. When I went in and spoke with the supervisor of the fast food joint I had boldness and told her I was a good worker but would not work on weekend or holidays because I had to visit my wife in prison in Phoenix. She agreed and I was employed making minimum wage in a place that gave me all the food I could eat on the days I worked.

Johna's words

When Ken told me about carrying the sign I again wondered what kind of man I was joined with. What was up with carrying a sign and looking like a homeless person. There was nothing I could do but pray and send him a care box. I had earned enough money, eleven cent an hour, plus some of my family had sent a $20 or $10 from time to time. So, I purchased all I could from the commissary and mailed a box of love to Ken. Much later he told me that the food allowed him to have a little extra for Maddie and himself and the stamps mailed allowed him to use his money for gas for the visit trip to Phoenix. I was concerned about Ken during these months. He was thin and seemed pale to me. One Saturday Ken didn't show up. By that time all the campus expected him and the word got to my CPO, which is the person in prison that works on an inmates' behalf kind of like a case manger. She was always nice and truthful and for some reason was at work on that Saturday. She came to me mid afternoon on Saturday telling me that a hospital from Tucson called and Ken was very ill. He had surgery having a cyst removed from his lower spine. The absolute feeling of despair is one I've never before or since felt. There was nothing I could do to relieve Ken's pain or comfort him. I called Harold. Later that day the CPO allowed a phone call to the hospital .I called Ken who was very much "out of it" but hearing his voice helped. Harold talked with me on Sunday and he had learned that Ken was doing okay.

Ken talks about it

Basically I worked, read the Bible and prayed and visited Johna. I felt tired a lot and thought the stress was taking a toll on me. You can know God's power and relief if you have to or if you decide to be completely dependent on Him. On a trip home from the prison I stopped to put my remaining $8 in the gas tank and buy a hamburger. It was weird, I came out from the fast food and gas stop and walked around the car backwards and then saw the back tire was frayed with the steel belts showing. I got back into the car and said, "God you know I need help. There is no spare tire but your word promises that whatsoever we bind on earth shall be bound in heaven. And so I bind the air in that tire and it is not going to go flat and there will be problem on the way home. And God when I get to the tire man he will be amazed." I drove the speed limit home and a few days later, when Dad sent money for a couple new tires, I drove the car to the tire repair shop. As the man was replacing the frayed tire he asked, "Where did you drive this from?" And then he said, "There is no way you drove this from Eloy and let the car sit a couple of days and then drove it here. The air would not stay in this tire." Needless to say, I was high on Jesus all over again!

Another time God helped me was driving home on a Sunday night after visiting Johna and the car stopped running. I called Danny and he towed me home. The next day Danny sent a friend over who looked at the car and fixed it for $30. This opened the door for me to witness to Danny about Jesus as I thanked him. He hugged me and shared about the difficulties he was having in life. I prayed faithfully for him many years after we no longer had contact with him. Danny had cancer and I don't know what happened with him but I believe he had an opportunity to know God.

Money was tight as I paid for rent, utilities and restitution because of the damage to the face of the person in Nebraska. I was here in Tucson on probation. The little food I bought was mostly food that I could share with Maddie. But she was good at eating cereal and top ramen with a little bit of liver in it if there was money for that. We shared. Most importantly, I always had money to drive the weekend trips to Phoenix. Sometimes I had to take Maddie and we'd sleep in the truck stop where there was running water because of the lack of money, and other times I had enough money to drive back and forth both days so Maddie got to stay home and we slept in our bed. Maddie was a comfort always to me. At the truck stop she was a pillow for my head as well as a heater for warmth and a loving companion. A great sadness for me was the need to have Maddie put to sleep. I could have kept her but it put me at risk of having to use money for a court hearing or a fine and there was only enough money to live and to see Johna. I would do nothing that put my visits with Johna in jeopardy. I had promised Johna that I would be careful and always able to visit her. A neighbor had a dog that ran free in the neighborhood. This person summoned me to court saying Maddie had hurt her dog. The person did not show at court so there was no big issue, but I knew we were on a downhill slide. Danny's brother was at the house and often left the door and/or gate opened and Maddie was old and had become determined to hurt anything that came near the yard. She was not in her right mind. I just knew it was coming to be a problem that I could not afford. So, I called animal control and they put her down. I was so sad.

On the trips back and forth from Phoenix I would cry and pray. One of the mountains ranges looked to me like Jesus and I told God, "I see Jesus in that mountain range, where do you see Him."

He said, "Do you really want to know."

"Yes Father I really want to know."

"I see Him everywhere. I see him in every mountain, every hill, every pile of rock. Every forest, every tree, every stick of wood reminds of the cross. I SEE HIM EVERYWHERE." I cried the rest of the drive home. This was the beginning of writing of THE VIAL SO PRECIOUS.

The writing was important and I know that never would I have attempted to write but for Johna. She was educated and she thought my words were strong, interesting and good. She expected that I take hold of this gift. In fact, it was her encouragement that caused me to accept that God had given me the "gift of words". She helped me accept that God is creative and when He gives a gift like writing He is giving a good and beneficial gift that too is creative. She caused me to see myself differently.

One Thursday night when I went to bed there was pain in my lower back and buttocks. About midnight I awakened and could feel a large growth on the bottom of my spine and I could not walk and the pain was very bad. A few days before I'd had my hair cut at a shop and the man who cut my hair was named Shawn. When he heard I was new in town he gave me a card with a private phone number. I dragged myself, literally, across the rooms to the phone and called that number. It was Shawn's cell phone and he was at a party but would be right to the house to take me to the hospital. He and a couple of his friends, they were dressed in pink tuxedos and had been partying for a while, carried me to the car and then into the emergency room. Shawn stayed until they took me to surgery and he helped instruct the hospital to contact my Dad and Johna in prison. I have never hurt more than during those hours before being admitted into the hospital and in the few days after being discharged. The growth was big and left a hole that had to be filled with gauze a couple times a day. It hurt. I lost weight and felt very weak. The prison somehow let Johna call me in the hospital and her voice was music to me. Again I knew things would be okay and that I would be to the prison by the following weekend. You know I did go see her the weekend after the surgery. The mother of one of the women in prison had become a friend and a male friend of this family was going to the prison and invited me to ride along. It was so painful that I knelt in the front floorboard putting my head on the seat and Johna and I stood up during the entire visit. I didn't see her on Sunday but it was important that I not miss one weekend. It was important to her and it was important to me. I had set my face toward God to do all I could to be faithful and consistent in my love of God and of my Johna.

Johna's words

There were several very precise lessons for me during the prison year about control and the fact that really I was not the answer to anyone's need or problem. I had gotten into the legal mess primarily because of greed and the need to be the rescue for another person. This kind of Messianic complex is a problem! I can smile these days thinking about the lessons but back then they were painful. Of course the situation with Ken being so ill was an example. When Ken came on the weekend to visit me and was so ill I realized that his love for me was strong and stronger than that was his commitment to God. Ken was a strong man and he would do what he believed God expected of him. I had never been part of anything this consuming. Another example of how God taught me His sovereignty and my need to wait on Him was scary. In the first week of being in prison I had a dream. The dream was so upsetting that I woke up during it feeling anxious and with panic in my throat. The dream was simply about a man who came toward me and he was wearing black boots that were shined to a glossy black color. I'll tell you the dream was so real that as I write these words that feeling of awareness and panic returns to my throat. Months later, about eight to be exact, I was working in the lobby of the men's prison and a guard entered the washroom where the supplies for me were stored. It was during a Census Count and I was reading the Bible. I did not look up when I became aware of a person entering the small room, but I saw the black highly polished boots and I knew this was a situation of danger. The guard was an Officer that some of the women had complained about among themselves. He approached me saying something like, "Hey how are you? We are alone. Stand up and look at me." I stood and looked him in the eye and said, "In the name of Jesus leave me alone." He was paged and as he left the room he said, "This isn't over." I remember saying to God that He and I were partners because He loved me and had promised to walk through the consequences of past wrongs to a place of higher ground where He and I could work together without the drain of my sinful past. You may think this is weird but I really depended on God and refused to be afraid. This event occurred prior to the furlough and until I returned from the furlough there were many happenings on the campus that I simply didn't see. This event opened my eyes to the degree of inappropriate sexual exchanges between the guards and the inmates. After the furlough the Administrator and some of the counselors and CPO were interviewing inmates and when my turn came I was asked about any concern I held for the safety of the inmates. What an opening. I gave the statement of the exchange with this guard. The day before this interview I had heard a noise and explored it only to see this same guard involved in sexual activity with an inmate. The inmate and I had eye contact and I quietly walked away. Once this statement was made I worked to keep anxiety and fear from me. Within two weeks of the interview this guard and his buddies were transferred out of duty for the women's prison camp. I realized that if I would listen God would protect me and He would be faithful to create times and places for my voice to be heard. In God there is safety. So often in my past I had spoken when and what I wanted and in reviewing those times I came to realize that though I called myself an advocate I generally was speaking to draw attention and honor to myself. Another understanding about my complex of being the advocate and answer to the problems of others came as I watched the women in prison. When there was a crisis like a husband was without employment or a child was ill or the woman had to appear before the parole board there was an intense request for prayer and a crying out to God. However, when the crisis passed regardless of the resolution the woman no longer needed intense prayer and there was no regard given to the Bible. I found this confusing and frustrating. What sense was there in calling on God in the middle of a problem caused by me and then ignoring Him during the answer or resolution or days of life following the crisis? The women gave little consistent attention to God. I came to realize that all I could do was lift up the name of Jesus and the response to Him was not my responsibility. Again, I gained freedom and a sense of relief as I realized God was the answer and the work of Johna was not.

Ken's point of view

One of the things that concerned me for Johna during some of her months in prison was the burden she carried for her fellow inmates. At first it was great. Johna was praying for and with some of the women; however, it became such a burden that God brought words of instruction to me for Johna. There were words to remind her that Jesus is the Savior and our job is to lift up His name in what we do and say, but the response to Him is not our job. She would write about her concern. I recall one woman; maybe the woman's name was Amy. This young woman was married and in prison for a white-collar crime. The woman showed an interest in God but then became involved in a homosexual relationship. Johna was very concerned and it was from this situation that I wrote her the letter that is published as THE PARABLE OF THE FRUIT. As I prayed for Johna in her work with other inmates I realized she was assuming too much responsibility for their decisions. It is tough to bring Jesus to others who then refuse to accept or take hold of His grace. Eventually I asked Johna to let go of all her relationships in prison and rest in the fact that she had been faithful to speak Jesus and to pray for the women. Later Johna told me this was a relief to her as the women would only take from God but were unwilling to give back their love and their will to His way. It was difficult to speak with Johna about this kind of truth because she was very educated and I felt inferior but God dealt with me reminding me that He waited for me right where I left Him. And, you know I had generations of Christian heritage and upbringing and there is nothing, not even a degree in law that is as truthful and powerful as His word. So, I learned to trust that God would make me a husband fit for this wonderful woman He gave me.

Johna shares

Another special exchange with God in prison was about the cleaning of the men's lobby. It was hard work. Some days as I walked from the women's prison across the desert to the men's unit I prayed to God asking He be my helper. I know that sounds dumb and even then I'd think how stupid I was praying for help in scrubbing the tile floors of the large lobby. Yet, I had no one else and felt overwhelmed with the job. Remember, the good work would mean a time out of prison with Ken. Time after time I'd get there and the guard would remark, "Hey, I thought you'd already been here. It looks good." I believe the angels helped me.

Several times I was privy to the arrival of a load of men into the men's prison. It was awful. What kind of people have we become? I remember thinking that I was a sister to this population of people and always would bow myself before God asking He help me be more like Him and less like the criminal I had become. It was in these exchanges that I so acutely realized that I was the property, in the eyes of the world, of the federal government and yet, because of God's great love, I was not even a citizen of this world but of heaven. Sometimes I yearned for the day when Jesus and I would be face to face.

The big greyhound type bus and sometimes two would arrive and the guard would tell me to disappear. That meant that I was in the cleaning supply closet. That was okay because I always carried my Bible and would read. Generally these off loads of people would take about an hour. Here's what occurred. Guards would line up with rifles drawn in a manner that the prisoners who came off the bus would have to walk down the aisle between the rows of guards with guns. The prisoners looked dirty and tired and were chained arms and feet and it was always very quiet except for the clanging of the chains. I could not help but look out of the crack in the door seeing all colors and sizes of men being admitted into the medium secure prison for crimes they had committed. You know I reviewed many women's pre-sentencing reports and never was there a case where the person had not committed the crime. It amazed me at so many hurting people. When a load came into the men's prison it might be 60 men and then there were loads going out of the prison of about the same number. Of course these loads in and out happened on different days. A guard told me they randomly moved prisoners as a method of behavior control. It wasn't that the men were treated badly or deserved to out of prison that made me sad.

The reality of the fact that so many people break the law caused me to know that only God is the answer and yet we are so careful to speak only politically correct or socially acceptable answers and statements. We need God.

Ken's words

I cleaned the house really good and arranged to have a couple extra days off from work because Johna was coming home from prison for five days. I was so nervous. What if we had nothing to talk about and what if she didn't love me out of prison; however, I knew that God had given us to one another and it was important to be gentle and kind. I drove to the Federal Prison Camp arriving about 20 minutes early. I waited until 5 minutes of the hour and approached the office. I was informed that Johna would be brought down in a few minutes. As I waited for her I prayed that God would let her see me through His eyes. I reminded God that His love of me was great and that His plan for my life was awesome and that Johna needed to see some of that as we spent time together. They called me into the office and I signed papers. In those moments I was grateful to Victor, the federal probation officer, who had checked out our home and agreed it was a safe place for Johna. He had given me some ideas about what to expect at this time of checking Johna out. Then, there she was, my wife. We walked to the car, got into the car and drove out of the parking lot to the exit back onto the interstate. We laughed. We kissed a couple of times and we cried and declared this would be five days of happiness and thankfulness to God who always met our need. We had to be in Tucson by a certain time and check in with the probation officer. That was no problem and he was very nice. I was sweating as Johna and I approached our humble home. This was the place I had prepared for her. That night it was really cold and Johna had the good idea of taking the curtains off the windows that had blinds on them anyway and using the curtains for blankets. I could not afford the gas bill so there was no heat; however the electric bill was paid so we had lights and a microwave plus refrigerator. I had to work a couple or three days during the furlough. Johna was so timid. She stayed home and watched TV, which was a treat as we got the station of old movies. I bought a couple gallons; really, of ice cream and during those days she ate both gallons. I was glad. Johna was so thin. One day she came to the fast food joint for lunch. It was only a few blocks to walk but that was a big deal to Johna and she came about 2 p.m. and then just waited until I was finished working because the exposure of the world outside prison caused her anxiety. I was saddened that the experience of prison had such a strong impact on my wife who had much education and life experience but found it difficult to walk the streets alone fearing that something would happen and snatch her back into the prison. I was her hero and protector and, I must say, it was a role that built my ego and brought joy to my heart.

Johna's words

Ken was waiting for me. All the women cheered as I left the cellblock but my heart hurt. What if he didn't like this person that I had become? I was no longer Johna the risk taking, loud talking, aggressive person that knew no pause. I needed Ken and without Jesus I was nothing. He smiled. We signed the papers and everyone was sweet. I thought of the respect Ken had earned from the guards and how they always allowed him to bring in his Bible and manuscript and never unless there was a new guard was I strip searched after a visit although that was the standard procedure. Ken was respected. We left. It smelled different and I rolled the car window down so the air of freedom could enter the car. The window didn't stay down long because in February the air is cool even in Arizona. I felt uncertain about whether to touch him but he put his hand on my head and prayed. I'll never forget this sweet prayer asking God to take anxiety and fear and to give us days of happiness and freedom and to remind us of the great love we held for one another. I hugged Ken. In case you haven't realized it, I love Ken. We kissed and we laughed. Then we talked and talked. It seemed as time flew and we were checking in with Victor the federal probation officer who was really nice, and then we were driving into the yard of the house Ken had sacrificed and rented so I could spend time with him.

The house was clean. It was cold but it smelled and looked and felt like Ken. To this day I have not experienced greater joy that the first night of the furlough. We made sweet love; however it is the holding and praying and sweet words of comfort that broke the case around my heart. Ken had to work a few days. When he left I was filled with panic, but he left ice cream and there were old movies and then I thought to call the Salvation Army asking for utility help for Ken, and you know what, they helped. The gas wasn't on before I left back to prison but

Ken had a month of gas paid and I was so happy that he was warm during those cool days of March. I went to the fast food place where Ken worked and as I walked the blocks between his house and the restaurant I would have turned back because of the great panic in my throat but for the knowledge that Ken waited for me. In the free world I felt exposed and vulnerable and afraid. When Ken came around the counter to greet me he seemed surprised by my tight hug and request for assurance that "everything is okay."

The days of the furlough quickly ended. When we reached the exit back to the prison Ken pulled into a scenic view spot. He told me that he was dealing with rage and asked that I pray for him. Never had I prayed publicly but here was my sweet husband confessing a weakness of character and expecting that I pray release and healing. So, I laid hands on Ken and declared that he was free of anger and then I prayed words of thanksgiving to our gracious Lord who is the deliverer of all pain. During our days in Colorado I had a glimpse of the anger residing in Ken and you know since the day of prayer on the way back to prison there has been no sign of rage or great anger in Ken. God touched Ken and I knew He had. So, we returned to prison full of God's peace and excited that little time remained before we were released to one another with the goal of lifting up the name of Jesus every day of our lives.

The days of prison after the furlough were strange and sometimes I still think about them and know that I lack complete understanding of the lessons to be learned from the events of those days. For example, one night a noise awakened me about 3 in the morning. When I stood at the cell door I realized many women were awake and wandering the cellblock. One woman told me to go look out the windows from the other side of the cellblock. I went and saw many guards and a long line of women chained hands and feet walking out of the camp. My Hispanic friend, a three-year plus inmate told me that some of the women were being moved and it was a way to control the inmates. I will never forget the sound of the guards yelling orders and the dragging chains as the women walked out of the camp. Some of the guards formed a line with guns drawn that the women walked in front of as they passed out of the yard. These women did not have time to gather their belongings or say good-bye to other inmates. They were ordered out of bed, to dress and to leave within a short period of time. My heart hurt and I prayed. It would have been good to say good-bye, God touch and bless you, but in truth I'll never see those women again and I missed some opportunities to speak Jesus. It was a powerful lesson.

The first lightning storm during the days of prison taught me about a belief held by some of the inmates. As the rain fell and the lightning grew a group of women moved cell-to-cell telling the inmates to quickly cover their mirrors and windows with either a towel or blanket. The mirror was not glass but aluminum like substance that slightly distorted the reflection. However, these women were serious and I made no noise of protest as they moved with authority and a swiftness that caused coverings to be in place before the storm really took hold. At a later time I learned that this group believes there was a power in the lightning that could enter the mirror or window and cause harm to the entire group of people residing in the dwelling place. Well, I think that is strange; however, it opened the door to talk about God who is greater than the lightning or the storm and who in fact is the author of such events. I found those kinds of exchanges fascinating and day-by-day I grew to love our God more and more.

One kind of special event happened for me while in prison. There are a lot of these kinds of events but I had a toothache and in fact that tooth has recently, 2/2002, started giving me some trouble again. I am in prison and my tooth hurts a lot. There is no good remedy except God. I thought of the passage of scripture in Ephesians where it reads, "But God, in His great wisdom..." So, I prayed and you know that tooth stopped hurting. Each time a pain would come in the tooth I refused to tell anyone. I didn't tell Ken or other inmates nor did I go to the medical call, I told God and every time it stopped hurting immediately. I admit that I've been reluctant to have it looked at since prison because He has always taken care of that pain.

This reminds me of medical call. One day I sat on the bench and watched the large number of women respond to the medical call. My heart hurt. These women would go for any medication. A popular and easy medication to get was a pill for constipation and many women had a large supply of this medication. Any kind of painkiller was popular and you could trade favors for even aspirin. I made it a point to avoid going to the medical call. When we were at Harold's before prison days, Ken took me to some relatives where they were working cattle. On that day I was stung by a bee and did not have my kit that I needed because of an acute allergy to bee stings. As my finger swelled and I felt my throat filling up I told Ken I'd been stung. He and his uncle, a very sweet man named Merle, put their hands on me, and Ken prayed. You know what, the swelling and the filling in my throat stopped and all I had was a little red spot. Well, I was stopped in my thoughts, feelings and words.

Months later on the prison compound I was stung by a bee. As panic filled my thoughts and my finger began to swell I closed my eyes and recalled the day on the farm when Ken and Merle prayed for me. The swelling stopped and again I had a little red spot. God's protection is big enough for all our little aches and pains and you know what, it is big enough for the big hurts too.

Once I returned from the furlough it was as if my eyes were opened. I know some of what I saw in the last few months of incarceration had been happening regularly before that time, but I didn't see it. It is my position that God protected me and I say, "Thanks God." In the weeks after furlough I saw more homosexual activity than I can even speak about and I think some of that is because a younger and more aggressive group of women were brought onto the compound. Always I thank God for His kindness in placing me in a camp where the average age of the inmate was 32 years and that He maintained that status until the last weeks of my time in prison. The younger women were very drug involved so more drug activity was on the campus and they were somewhat gang related so the talk and associations on the compound changed. The younger women were quick to engage in one and then another homosexual relationship and they were bold and public about these relationships. In the mix of this the interactions between the guards and the inmates became more and more sexual and inappropriate. There was no safety on the compound except in Christ. It was in this context that I first had an encounter with the angels of God who continue to be partners in my life in Christ.

Ken and I experienced angels again in our work with Casa Gloriosa; but my first encounters with them were in prison. I can't relate these facts about or exchanges with the angels to you because I really don't know how. I do know that again I was changed and it was good. I want to say that I would not trade the days of prison. I learned a lot about last chance people, about God and about me and I came to rely, to depend and to expect God. It was a good year in my life. God took my crime and my wrong and turned it inside out into usefulness. I stand amazed and grateful.

Very soon after furlough was Valentine's Day. Ken was allowed, the guards really had a sense of trust and respect for him, to bring into the prison at visit time two large valentine's, two plastic wine glasses and some chocolate candy. He sat up the table before I was admitted into the visit room. We had a soda from the machine. My heart was undone. That visit morning few, maybe one or two, women had visitors so Ken and I had a great deal of privacy. It was so helpful to have this private exchange so soon after the furlough. Ken has an ability to make the most out of every difficult situation and he always brought surprise and fun to the prison visits. Valentine's Day in prison was one of my most special days.

Ken shares

The days of prison were some of the most difficult in my life. Johna was apart from me and yet I remained steadfast and faithful to her and to God. They were good months that developed character and caused me to know that I had set my face like flint toward God and that nothing could make me look away from Him. At the end of those days I knew that God in me was strong and that nothing but my lack of faith could cause a falling away from God. I rejoiced. It was good when the prison days ended but they were days of growth and wonder. I remain thankful for being part of that experience.

Johna's words

My friends had a farewell for me on the evening before the departure from prison. The black women sang and sang and I was blessed. One woman asked me to pray and another told me, "I'd never thought of you as an educated uppity white woman. You were our friend." Everything but my Bible, the letters from Ken that I had not mailed back to him and the pictures I gave to the women. When you are released you can have a new dress and shoes from Penney's valued at $50 or you can have the money. I opted for the money that would be mailed to me along with the $32 in my prison account. Sleep was far from me that evening and I really didn't try to get much. I stayed outside until the guard called to lock the cellblock and then I stayed with a group of women and I talked more that night than previously. In fact, the women asked questions and I honestly answered and, for the most part, glory and honor was given to God.

Ken had become a symbol of hope and example to many of the women and we re-read some of his letters. For the last couple of months there was a reading of some of his daily letter to as many as 25 women. Ken always wrote about God and the women were always eager to hear. So, that night I asked them, as a group, if they knew God and told them the plan of salvation. There was respect among us, the last call for everyone to return to her cell was made, and then I was alone in my cell. As I reviewed this year I knew that God had taken my wrongs and my willingness to be His person and in that mix He had anchored my soul in Christ Jesus. Nothing would sway my love for Him, and in that, the next phase of life would be okay.

On the morning of May 12th I stepped outside the front prison door, waved farewell to the group standing inside and stepped into the taxicab headed toward the bus station. Ken could pick me up and take me to the halfway house but he had to pick me up from the bus station. It was a strange taxicab ride and I felt anxious and uncertain. At the station the cab driver reminded me the prison paid the fare and that I was to be on the 11 a.m. bus to Tucson. He left. I looked for Ken. The bus would leave in 15 minutes and there was no Ken. Finally I asked at the counter if there was another bus station and sure enough there was and the person took pity on me and called asking for Ken Reeves.

When Ken answered the page he assured me he'd be at the station in 30 minutes. So I waited and the bus to Tucson left and then suddenly Ken was there full of smiles and hugs. He reminded me that we had hours before I had to check in at the halfway house. I was glad that Ken had moved into the neighborhood of the halfway house.

Chapter Three: Released from Prison

Ken's point of view

She is going to be released from prison. Not one day early. I had always believed and had cried out many times to God that Johna's release would be early; however the year had passed and she was going to be released into a halfway house. I didn't understand what caused Johna to be reluctant and upset about this release. So, I walked by the halfway house several times and prayed. I sensed this would be a difficult transition time for both Johna and me. She would have to be in the house for one month and perhaps two months. So, I decided to move into a mobile home park located directly behind the halfway house. The managers were really nice people and had a ministry to people being released from prison. They gave me the best deal possible and I thanked Danny for his many kindnesses and rented a 10 by 50 mobile home. It was a good thing that Dad visited in June and he and I painted the entire home and laid a new carpet in the front room. Later I learned this mobile park was one of the worse for crime, drugs and child abuse in the county. The day for Johna's release arrived and eventually we made it back to Tucson. She was anxious but I would not take her to the halfway house even one hour early. She could go the next day to the fast food place and get a job and as I left her at the halfway house we agreed I'd stop in about 10 a.m. the next day. That would give her time to learn the rules and be ready to walk the 6 miles to the food place for a job interview. She could start that afternoon shift if she wanted and the halfway house agreed.

Johna's point of view

The Director of the halfway house astonished me. She talked vulgar and flirted with some of the inmates about an advertisement she was going to do for pay. She was dressed sensually and the looks among the inmates let me know they thought they had her number. I felt unsafe. It was 9:30 a.m. and I'd been waiting since 8 o'clock for the interview I was supposed to have with her and in fact was told that I had to have before I could leave the property. Ken came but I could not leave with him. A couple of days passed and nothing was done except to sign some papers and be told there was a law firm that would interview me and I was expected to take the job because 75% of whatever I made during the two months at the halfway house was rent for staying there. I called the probation officer who had already met Ken for the approval for the furlough. He agreed to come see me the next day. Ken took my application, he was allowed an hour visit each day, to his employer and came back to tell me I could start immediately and that I was assigned to work his shifts. The meeting with the Director, the Probation Officer and myself was awful. I learned that there would be no early release like I had been promised. I was told do one month there successfully and the second you will be out on probation. The PO argued on my behalf but the Director told us that the pay for a federal inmate was the highest pay received and unless another woman was released from the federal prison she had no intentions of an early release for me. The PO privately told me there was nothing he could do except try and have me sent back to prison. He was successful however in getting me released to the fast food job. So, I decided that seeing Ken from 1 p.m. when we left walking the 6 miles to work where we worked until midnight or 1 a.m. and then walked back to the halfway house was better than prison. I was reminded that God is the protection and the answer to situations both in prison and out of prison.

Ken tells about it

Working at the fast food place was tough on Johna but it was better than staying an extra hour at the halfway house. I started walking around the place several times in the morning before she was released and then during the early morning hours after she returned to the compound. A guard told me, "We watch them all day and night." And I replied, "And I'm watching you." That's how we felt about that place. It was awful. But then Dad came and as always that helped. Johna was then able to get out of the place about 10 a.m. and return only after our work shift. During the days Dad was here we fixed up the mobile home, ate good food and again spent lots of time in the Word of God. July 12th finally arrived and the Probation Officer came on the compound, I think, to make sure Johna was released. She now was on probation for 3 years or until her restitution was paid.

Johna's words

I called my Mother during the first days of being out and in the halfway house. She accepted the collect call but I knew that we still had some work to do before our relationship was restored. Knowing that I'd caused so much pain and that there was no reason or defense all I could do was resolve in Christ to be faithful, truthful and allow His way to work in my life. In that position I felt that God would work on my behalf for restoration.

Working at the fast food place was great and it was awful! Ken was funny and everyone liked him. The manager told us that during the months Ken had been employed the profit was up 25% and the management believed it was Ken's work and attitude and impact on both customers and fellow employees. They wanted him to get into the "management track". The kids that worked there were fun and it was good to spend all the hours of every day with Ken. That was great plus we were in very good physical shape. After 6 weeks we bought bikes and had a lot of fun biking all over town. We biked to a church about 8 miles from the house that was known as a place where people coming out of prison could feel comfortable.

Ken's words

The first Sunday we attended Johna turned pale as we entered into the congregation of about 300 people. She was very nervous and felt awkward. It was a good church. There was a sense of unity and outreach and kindness. Our friend, Randy, who lived at the mobile home park introduced us to this church. To this day I don't think I've ever known a person who loved the church more than Randy. It was a good place for us to attend. We were not directly involved but rather allowed to watch the interactions of God's people. It was in this church that I played my last organized sport, baseball. The team was fun. We won the citywide championship. Looking back, the injury to my leg caused by a simple slide into home plate took months to heal and should have been a clue that something was not exactly right with my health.

Johna talks

Working at the fast food place was a good experience for me. It was hard work and we had to wear a uniform that declared we were employees of the joint, and we were by far the oldest people working there and we made minimum wage. One day walking to work in the hot sun, remember it can easily be 102 degrees at 1 p.m. in Tucson, a bird flew over us and pooped in my hair. Ken laughed until he saw my face. I was getting tired of this work. Later that day working hard I took a few minutes out and sat down in the back away from the customers. It wasn't break time but I wanted a break! Ken quietly spoke into my ear, "Johna come on, get back to work, you are a Reeves." He smiled and patted my back but he was serious. What in the world was his problem? How could he talk to me like that and then I thought, "Johna, you have never be exact." Well, as I diligently worked the rest of the shift I talked with God about my compromises, and doing just about enough and making rational defenses for doing it my way, and I repented. This lesson sticks in my thinking. God wants us to be exact. When He asks us to do something he will show the way and He expects us to obey His way. He really expects us to be and act His way, and then I was excited. If God expects us to be exact that means we are capable of such a lifestyle. What an adventure and what a challenge. There is no way to live in this manner but with the help of the Holy Spirit.

Ken tells about it

Closing the fast food restaurant about midnight we biked home carrying again the leftover food on our backs. It was a good evening. We were on the way home and we were together. We stopped for the red light and then biked across Oracle on Glenn Street.

Suddenly a car was following us and someone from the car yelled out at us. Johna looked back at me. "Don't say anything to them, don't answer them, act like they aren't here," I spoke with authority and calmness. There was a driver and a person in the passenger front seat, but it was the passenger in the back seat with the rifle pointed at us that caused me to think our life was over. I recall praying, "God, take us both. Don't leave us crippled or raped or hurt or alone." Later Johna told me she too prayed this prayer. The car pulled off the road between us and had caused Johna to stop biking. Again I called her name and we maintained eye contact believing that we were breathing our last breath. Suddenly the man with the rifle that was trained on us laughed. It was a evil nasty laugh and he said, "Hey I was just kidding, I was just kidding. Let's go, let's go." The car quickly peeled away from us leaving Johna and me smiling. We embraced and thanked God for the angels that once again protected us. To this day, I am confident that the man saw our angels and wanted no part of them. By the way, one of my angels is named Chuck. I've written a poem about Chuck, my beloved angel.

Johna shares

The food we carried home in the backpack was the leftover of the fast food joint that the manager told us we could have. Let me tell you, Ken is really a good manager of money. We lived on nothing. Consider that about 75% of what I was making went to pay restitution and we were then making minimum wage; however we had need of nothing. In fact, living at the mobile home park among very poor, some mentally ill and other recent prison released people we were grateful for the blessings in our life. Ken always will give his last dollar or best shirt to a needy person. So, it was with great joy that he'd carry, six miles, a heavy backpack of leftover food so we could bless the people of the park.

Ken's words

Alfred became my helper. After a while the mobile home owners asked me to manage the park because the couple that had done the work was moving to another job. Alfred had a drug problem. He was a crack head but he was really a good guy. One day I handed him the keys of the park as part of a statement of my faith in him and the need for him to help me with a project. It was fun to watch him strut so proud was he to be part of the boss. It made me think of how God always gives us another opportunity. Years later it was Alfred's brother who assisted us, in his job, to get the railroad disability and again I was reminded of how nothing is coincidental.

Johna's words

Ken is a man's man. There was this old guy, Clem, that had been a Sgt. Major or something in the military and I know he was a big deal because of old paperwork we saw and his monthly military pension. When Clem was sober he was striking and he had a marvelous artist talent. Ken talked about his "bearing and grace of a gentleman" when he was sober and Ken loved this old man. Clem was mostly not sober however and in fact I know of two times Ken rescued him. Ken is good at rescuing last chance people and in those days of mobile park living I got to watch my husband be Jesus over and over to the ugly people. One time Clem called Ken asking for a ride from a bar. Ken took me with him that time. I think Ken wanted me to become educated in the rescuing of these kinds of people. Clem was very drunk, had soiled himself and was crying happy to see Ken. With tenderness and respect Ken cleaned him up, took him home and put to bed. The other time was even more dramatic. Alfred, oh what can I say about Alfred, came running and yelling to Ken that Clem was dead. Ken ran across the mobile home park and found Clem, sure enough, almost dead. Ken had to resuscitate Clem. Imagine giving this kind of attention to a person drunk, slobbery and unconscious. Well, the ambulance arrived and they let Ken into the vehicle to escort dying Clem to the VA hospital. Now, during the ride and in the emergency room Ken prayed and as Clem came back around he prayed the prayer of salvation. Clem recalls this experience as having Ken in his ear telling him that he was going to die and needed Jesus. Last chance people are precious.

Ken's words

Black Pearl, the name we fondly bestowed on a woman with about six kids who moved into the mobile home park. She was my buddy. She always smiled and gave us a lot of sweet potato pie. It was good talking with her about Jesus and she knew of His great love. However, all her children were drug involved, in prison or looking to avoid being seen by the police who often patrolled the park. I never could understand how she knew of God's love so much and yet never experienced it. I wonder about her.

Johna shares

One of the fun things in our life during this phase was the old girls. The old women have always loved my husband. I think partly because Ken has always been bigger than life and in that you feel safe. As the manager of the park all the old ladies knew and loved him. So, every Thursday night we all had dinner with Esther who insisted on being the cook and then we played games for a couple of hours. It was fun to see these old people respond to attention and to reminisce about the days of joy and family.

Ken's words

The job at the fast food place was taking its toll and Johna was looking for a better job. My heart went out to her as she applied in many places only to be turned down because of her felony status. She was on federal probation and the terms of the probation required disclosure of that status. So, she was quickly getting called to interviews but just as quickly being turned down. The amount of restitution required a higher level of income in order to pay it off in the three years of assigned probation. I believed it was most necessary for her to become involved in a different work environment. Since her release she was full of anxiety and sometimes-panic attacks. For example, there were times she'd cry and talk with me about her feeling of being watched and concerned of being put back in prison. It was like she thought that everyone who looked at her knew that she was a felon and thought she deserved that position. In truth there were no people holding this kind of opinion and that concerned me for Johna. I would wonder about her being so freaked after prison and yet she seemed to have dealt with the prison months with calmness and dignity. In this period of time Prison Fellowship contacted Johna and it might have been possible for her to be employed with the national office. I felt really strongly that this would not be the right employment situation. So, I told her that if she worked for Prison Fellowship she would develop a reputation of being the ex-con. It helped my point that Randy, our friend out of prison for maybe 5 years, still talked the language and identified with the prison lifestyle. For example, he was going to "put 'em on front street" to get to the truth and he often, in the introduction of himself, shared his ex-con status. So, Johna agreed to not explore Prison Fellowship employment.

Johna's words

Another interview and I wondered what's the use. This must have been the 10th time that a job had set up an interview and it was another job for which I was very qualified; however, they would not hire me because, oh yes, I'm a felon. It made me sick.

Ken agreed to bike with me to the interview which was about 7 miles from our house. I recall tying my long grayish hair back, wearing one of the only outfits I had from my before prison days and that was a pair of white cotton pants and a blue and white cotton sweater. And, I did have new tennis shoes. The trip to the shelter where I was interviewing took longer than we thought so we arrived about 10 minutes late and I was sweating just a little. However, the newly hired Assistant Director and her group of other professional staff interviewed me. I was in that place that it really didn't matter, so I talked freely and with creativity as we talked about how to manage hurting children. The interview was positive and I did not fill in the blank on the application that asked about felony status. Two days later I was called and offered a job as the Social Work Supervisor for one of the oldest shelters for abused and neglected children in the United States. Within a few weeks of being employed we were able to move out of the mobile home to a little house near the shelter. Ken was working with Randy in roofing and carpenter work.

This was the first professional employment I had experienced since becoming a Christian. Ken and I prayed a lot for me, for the employees and for the children. It was a wonderful five years. Some of the events were especially sweet for me. During the entire time I was the supervisor we required only five children to be removed for misbehavior and most of those children had been in care at the shelter previously. A shelter is where children who have been treated badly and therefore often act in hurtful and difficult ways are placed by the state or by parents. One reason we were able to keep the children is because there were some marvelous people hired by the Assistant Director and myself. Rosie had been there for a long time as the Medical Director and there is no one better than Rosie with the kids and in understanding their issues both medically and developmentally. Rosie was always a person I could talk with and for whom I have great respect. Stacey was a childcare worker and I recall the first time I saw her. She was holding a baby, rocking with her foot another in a carrier, giving yet a third a bite of food and a smile and talking on the phone. When I entered the house she smile and indicated she'd be with me in a minute. After a while we promoted her to social worker and she was great. Her first encounters with the clients were full of judgment and she told me this was not the job for her. She agreed to stop trying so hard and to pray for the clients more, and of course she became one of the best. Ken and I were part of her marriage and she remained like a daughter even calling from Texas where she completed her Master's in Social Work. It was a difficult thing to speak at her funeral when she was killed in a car accident. I really think Stacey was the most pure person I have ever known and I think God spared her from too much pain. Jeanne, the Executive Director, ran the agency with efficiency and compassion. I recall the feelings the day I asked to talk with her. In the two months I'd worked for the agency no one asked about the blank line inquiring about my felony status but I had been fingerprinted and thought any day they would return with the big disclosure. So, here I came to talk with her. She listened; she thanked me for my candor and asked to talk with me the next day after she consulted with the agency attorney. That night I told Ken if they were uncomfortable with me working there I would resign because of the respect I held for the agency and people. Ken agreed. Jeanne was really nice about this situation, put a note in my personnel file in a sealed envelope and told me she appreciated my work. She remains a friend.

We had not been living in the new place too long when Randy called me telling me that Ken was ill. I went home. Randy had basically carried Ken off the roof of the house they were working on and then into our home. Ken lay on the floor on his back groaning. It was frightening. As I applied a cool rag to his head I watched the muscles in Ken's back, stomach, and legs contract. I called a friend in the medical profession who of course thought he should go to the emergency room but also recommended he drank Gatorade or Pedialyte. I purchase some of both and stayed awake a long time that night watching and praying for Ken. The next day he agreed to not work for several days and to look for another kind of employment. The nagging concern that Ken was ill lingered in my mind.

There are a couple happenings during these years at the shelter that definitely helped form my spiritual resolve. A four-year-old boy was admitted into the shelter and he was a biter. He bit everyone that came near him and he bit until there was blood and there needed to be no provocation. After a few days the staff requested his discharge. I agreed to meet with them the next day. That evening as I shared with Ken his quick response brought a feeling of impatience in my mind. Ken said, "Pray for him." This child had been in so many placements and rejected so many times. So I went to the shelter and stood at the bedside and prayed for this child. God knew and surely we could work through this problem. The next afternoon at the meeting the day shift worker reported there had been no biting. The group decided to keep him some more days. You know, I only shared with Ken about the prayer time, but that little boy did not bite during the remaining months he was in shelter and he became "one of the favorite kids." This was one of the first times I thought about the verse that says the angels of the children report to God every day. It makes me careful about the treatment I give and endorse being given to children.

Another time I was called by a worker, about 10:30 p.m., saying that the kids were rioting in the building of the older youth. That building held about 18 kids and back then we had kids from 8 to 12 years of age placed in it. Working with this group of children was always challenging. So, I grabbed on some clothes and Ken and we were at the shelter in a few minutes. There was a riot of sorts. The kids were all up yelling, running and throwing whatever they could get their hands on. For a minute I watched the children and I knew Ken was silently praying. One boy, he was about 9 years old and cross-eyed, was leading the noise and confusion. I asked Ken to pick him up removing him to his room. Once that child was out of the way everyone calmed down, followed instructions in the clean up and went to bed. I found Ken sitting on the bed holding this boy who was sleeping as Ken softly sang to him. It was years, about 8 in fact, that I saw this youth at a Child Protection Service office. He ran to me and immediately asked, "How is your husband, Ken?" He told me that he had never felt so safe as the night Ken picked him up, prayed for him and then sang him to sleep. We continue to pray for this young man who has experienced much pain and rejection.

It was Fourth of July, in the first year of employment at the shelter, and we gave time off to all the workers in the building for the older children and the Assistant Director, her husband Don, Ken and I became the childcare workers. Four people with about 18 kids! It was a fun day and I recall Ken falling, fully dressed, into a kid's pool much to the amusement of the children. All day he entertained the children. At one point I needed to get ice from the building. When I entered the front door it was as if shadows moved and I was very afraid. I walked to the back of the building saying out loud, "In the name of Jesus I am okay and nothing in this building can hurt me." When I returned to the group I privately told Ken. He and our friend, Don, went to the building walking through it praying. I am confident that these kinds of prayers allowed us to be successful with children that really were challenging, and I believe this was training days for the eventual home for HIV infected people.

When we talk about shelter we have to speak about Andy. He was a gift to us and I knew that the day I hired him as social worker. He was a sponge, committed to learning how to positively impact children that were torn and discarded. Andy was always willing to try. He was newly married to Cindy. Andy had a way with the older kids. There was difficult to manage young girl that one day in anger yelled at Andy, "You are a bitch." All the kids became quiet watching to see what was going to happen to this girl.

With no apparent distress Andy replied, "Really. Hey, someone get me a dictionary." When the dictionary was brought to Andy he handed it to this girl and told her if he fit the definition she could call him a bitch every day.

After looking up the meaning of bitch the girl started laughing and read, "A female dog." The situation was diffused; the girl saved face and even apologized to Andy.

Ken shares

Cindy and Andy introduced us to a couple who were going into ministry and needed someone to live in their mobile home way out on the west side and the cost was $200 per month. Johna and I drove out there and immediately knew that, if possible, we would move. We had been living near the shelter but that area in the previous year had become known as "sugar hill" because of the flow of cocaine. It would be great to have some privacy and to pay less rent. Our finances were tight with most of Johna's income still going to restitution. I smiled about that, the first Christmas she worked at the shelter we were expected to go to the party at a nice Italian restaurant and we were so nervous.

What to wear? Johna had a black dress, very short, and an ostrich feather jacket so all she needed were high black heels. Somehow that outfit was stuck in with her few prior prison belongings. She pulled her hair up off her neck and looked good. So we went thrift store shopping with $25 to buy both of us shoes, and some kind of jacket for me that would be okay with my black dress pants and silk shirt. We prayed. The first store we visited had a dinner jacket, off white, late 1950's plus a pair of tie up black dress boots for me and a brand new pair of black heels for Johna and the cost was $24.95. We felt better. I asked Randy to give us a ride in his 1956 Cadillac recently repainted. And, we were off. When Randy let us out we looked at one another, smiled and straightening our shoulders entered the restaurant knowing we were subject to a few questions about the who and why of us. Every time I think of this situation I love Don all over again. He was the Assistant Director's husband and a well-positioned businessperson in town who became my great buddy. That night he was gracious and though he later denied knowing what he was doing he covered and smoothed every difficult question for us.

Johna's point of view

It was only a month that I had been employed for the shelter when a call from a prison in Tucson was placed to the social work supervisor of the shelter, and that was me. The request was for a person to come, as a volunteer, into the prison release facility and teach a parenting class. I agreed to "get back" with the prison official. I talked with Ken who thought it would be good for me to get involved in this volunteer work. When I called the probation officer he had no problem with me volunteering in the state prison but told me that would not happen because of my felony status. He agreed I could try and so I called back the prison official and gave my name, social security number and date of birth saying I'd be willing to teach the class. About three weeks later Joan, the prison person, called me and asked when I could start.

Ken's point of view

Johna asked about doing volunteer work in the Arizona state prison release center for women and immediately I knew this was a good deal for her. I promised Johna that I would lie on my face before God every hour she was in that prison doing volunteer work. Of course, God is smart and I didn't realize how many hours I would lay before God for my wife. Praying for Johna as she worked for God was a sweet experience. You know when she was in prison it seemed, sometimes, that we met in the spirit. I know that is strange, but we would write every day and those letters are evidence of times when she and I independently felt we connected. Praying for Johna as she was speaking truth in the prison was a similar experience for me. I saw her as God saw her, full of compassion and understanding and love for those incarcerated women.

I was proud of her that never in her prison work did she disclose her story. There was no need. She was doing the work to lift up the name of Jesus and not the story of Johna. I loved her in a new way.

Johna shares

It would, I think be good, if you could feel my emotions and think my thoughts the first time I went onto the state prison compound to teach a class. Here I was an ex-con still on probation going onto a prison compound to teach a group of women about parenting. And, I was going not as an ex-con or a Christian but as a social worker with expertise in teaching about children and parenting. I knew Ken was home bowed before God on my behalf praying that God would use this to touch incarcerated women and their children. It was a great class of 23 women in a too small room. The weeks passed quickly and the last, the 10th week, arrived. At the end of that class I told the women that we were finished with the class and I was pleased that all who started had completed the course. "Did anyone have a suggestion about how to close this time together?" I asked.

"Yes," a large African American woman said, "I know what we need to do." Without more explanation she came and stood before me. "Pray Mrs. Reeves. Pray for me." Now this was mysterious because in the 10 weeks I had been careful to share nothing personal and nothing about my belief and faith in Jesus Christ, and it caused a pause in me because the only person I'd prayed out loud with and for, previous to this date, was Ken.

"Okay," I timidly said and started to pray, "Oh God..."

"No, I mean really pray Mrs. Reeves. Like this." She put her arms up in the air with her hands spread. "Now you put your hands in front of mine and pray that God takes this demon of cocaine away from me. You know Him, so pray and I will believe."

Well, what can you do? I prayed with my eyes tightly closed and as that prayer ended and I opened my eyes I fell in love with the Holy Spirit all over again. Every woman was lined up waiting for a prayer. So started my volunteer time in prison and it lasted about a year. I was at least 15 hours a week in that state prison. There was no chaplain, no therapist and only one or two other programs for the women. I was called at all hours and for all kinds of needs and God healed the frayed edges of my heart as He used me to touch and pray with the women at this prison.

At the end of about one year of volunteer work the prison official asked me to do more work in the development of a curriculum to assist women to find employment. Ken and I talked about this opportunity and decided that I needed to share my felony status with the prison administration before accepting the volunteer position. The day I talked with the Administrator and the activity coordinator I again felt nervous but knew that if God wanted me in the prison He would work it out. I was given an Independent Contractor's card that actually allowed me in all the prisons in the State of Arizona if opportunity was presented. God is funny! So, I developed a curriculum and a graduate student assisted in teaching it to these women. Out of that I contacted the Prison Fellowship person whom I had known while incarcerated and we developed a plan for providing the services of Prison Fellowship to the then approximate 700 women in Pima County in prisons. So, I became the Prison Fellowship Coordinator for women in Pima County.

The work with Prison Fellowship causes me to mention Leigh Anne. She was an employee at the shelter. Her work ethic was exemplary and she was a quick study and willing to be the best for the children. She worked with all the groups of children but I most recall her work with the infants and particularly with the drug exposed babies. She would sing and hold them and work with them and it was fun to watch her. I recall Rosie and I speaking of a feeling of relief that Leigh Anne was assigned this special group of children. So, I made an assumption that she was a Christian and invited her to be part of the first weekend Prison Fellowship retreat I was facilitating.

Leigh Anne accepted the invitation to be part of the weekend retreat held at a newly opened state prison for women where about 500 women were placed on the compound. Ken and I were part of a church and recruited the other 21 women who would go into the prison that weekend with me. One young woman, Sandy, was the music person and she is awesome and we really worked well together. The topic of the seminar was "Loving Others" and it was my first in prison weekend retreat.

Friday night about 90 inmates showed up for the meeting. As Sandy lead the women into worship I was completely undone and took a few minutes in the hallway thanking God that in His grace He allowed me this experience. When I stepped back into the front of the room I looked across the women. To me it was a crowd of beautiful faces. As the women sang I noticed a pink mist that joined the women who had come into the prison with me. I merely breathed in knowing that His Spirit was big in that place. As the weekend continued additional women attended and some, I know, found God in a real way because they continue to serve Him.

Leigh Anne later told me that she was not serving God though her background was religious; however, in the prison she reconnected with God. Truly, Leigh Anne came into the heart of Ken and myself like a daughter and now her daughter, Jenna, is one of the most precious people in our life. When we feel tired, ready to give up or just beat up with all the pain of others we see Jenna and are ready to be all we can be in Christ Jesus. She is pure, smart and she loves us and especially Ken. It is joy to watch this beautiful child love people living with AIDS.

In the meantime some really awesome stuff was happening at the shelter and Ken and I were moving ahead on paying off my restitution. It was in this time frame that Harold, Ken's dad, fell in love with Lois and the marriage date was set. Ken and I must attend that function in North Platte, NE. We contacted Ken's probation officer in Pima County and were given the go ahead to attend that function. During the wedding ceremony, which was beautiful, I saw Ken's daughters and that was special; however, a probation officer who had known Ken for a long time and did not like him had issued a pick up order on Ken. So, the police arrested and jailed Ken immediately following the ceremony.

Ken shares

In the days we had lived with Dad prior to the incarceration of Johna we met a couple, Dallas & Marge, who are forever a part of our lives. The best memory of Dallas was an evening when Dad's church was reading the Bible through and Johna and I had taken the late night shift. Dallas came into the church and was so caught in the word that he stayed, cried and we prayed together and became forever friends. This couple was at the wedding, privy to the arrest and went with Johna back to Dad's house. Johna often has spoken about Dallas sitting up the night talking with her about God and the facts of our life and God's presence in it. After we were settled with Johna working at the shelter Dallas and Marge sent their three children to spend a month with us in Tucson. We love those kids. Megan came and worked with us much later when the shelter for HIV infected people was established and she holds a very special place in our hearts. The Wilkies are people we can always count on and much later I told Johna that she could count on Dallas.

Johna's point of view

I could hardly believe that Ken was arrested. And, the probation officer had stated that he was dangerous and if he resisted the arresting officer was to "shoot to kill". When I read that in the order there came an anger in me that helped me get through the next hours of this ordeal. At one point I thought Ken would merely have to do the time because there seemed to be no relief. There was a meeting in the Judge's chambers. We hired an attorney thanks to Ken's aunt who has always loved him a lot. At this meeting was Ken, me, Ken's attorney, the Prosecuting Attorney, Ken's dad, Dallas and Marge and the Judge as well as the probation officer. At one point the Judge insisted on a settlement and told us that he felt the system had been prejudicial and that there was wrong dealing with Ken but that to sort it all out Ken would have to sit at Kearney in the prison awaiting a trial. In the conference room I offered to call people in my family to see if there was a possibility of money but suggested this was not likely due to my past lying and deceitful taking of money from family members. Harold talked about getting a loan. The Prosecutor told us that $5000 would be acceptable and would end all Ken's legal issues and without that he would be taken to prison to await trial. We had about an hour to respond. To this day I believe that had Ken gone to prison a couple of things would have happened. One, it is likely that he would have been vindicated in that he was paying restitution and following the requirements of the State of Arizona and the probation officer had a long held grudge against Ken that resulted in wrong doing. Secondly, I think Ken would have become ill in the prison and our spirits would have been broken. Dallas and Marge without much ado produced $5000 and paid for Ken's release. We owe them so much more than money. What can you do in the face of this kind of debt? Pray that God blesses them, and so we pray. Ken and I flew home as scheduled relieved of one more burden.

About this time in our marriage I really wanted to file for a bankruptcy and be relieved of some of the debts we held and especially some that I had acquired prior to marriage. Ken however would not agree. We had some good talks about this difference in thought and Ken was right. We made the debts, we owed them and we needed to pay.

You know it took about 12 years to get out of debt to everyone except my family. I believe a day will come when that debt too is paid. You see, even while in law school I was a schemer and deceiver. My Mother and Aunt gave me large amounts of money because they believed I was ill. That was a lie. I was not ill.

The three years of probation passed and every month about 75% of my income was paid toward restitution and the last month of probation the last payment was made and I as free. It is interesting to me that every day of the sentence had to be completed. There was a need in Ken and me, and I hate to admit it, to have external boundaries. In those years he and I developed with the help of the Holy Spirit internal controls. There was a time that all I knew were two absolutes. One absolute in my life was that GOD IS and the second was that I would do sex with no one other than my husband. Over the years God has set other absolutes and the lines of our life connect between those making a filter that keeps us safe. It is a good to live a righteous life.

I have one last statement about the years of working at the shelter. During perhaps the third year a family of children was admitted to the shelter by the state of Arizona. These children were difficult; however endearing. I really liked their dad but he was not able to provide for them and had been abusive and very neglectful. One day the dad, Charles, came into my office telling me that the state was going to severe his parental rights and he wanted to give his children, at least his daughter, to me. Well, that was not possible for many reasons. However, I loved these kids and especially Heather. She had lived at the shelter almost a year, off and on, and the state thought she was headed to a residential treatment center although she was only about 5 years old year old. Heather was a very strong willed child, a survivor and able to protect herself and her three brothers. She had an older and two younger brothers. The state workers and parents signed a form allowing us to take the children in the shelter to a community church. Ken and I habitually took the older children to a church where the music, guitars and drums, really held the attention of the children. On this Sunday about 14 kids went in the shelter van with us. Ken sat on one end of the pew and 13 kids were between him and me and then Heather sat on the end next to me. I'll never forget her blue silk dress and black patent leather shoes and her square sturdy body. I loved her. The music was very good and the pastor stepped to the microphone at the end of it saying, "There is people here today that hurt. If you hurt come forward I want to pray for you." The noise of the 13 kids caused my attention to center away from Heather. She hit my leg and by the time I looked in her direction she was halfway down the aisle going to the front. I looked at Ken and he winked. Heather stood at the end of about 4 people waiting for prayer. She was on tiptoe leaning forward waiting for pastor's attention. Eventually he came to her and said into the microphone, "Little girl, what it is that I can pray for you?"

Heather into the microphone in a strong voice said, "You said you'd pray if we hurt. I hurt. Pray for me." I've never witnessed before or since a group of people, that day about 350, lay aside their personal agendas and reach toward God on behalf of another with such intensity. It was a holy moment. The pastor prayed for her and Heather returned to her seat and hugged me.

When we returned to the shelter Ken told me that we needed to speak with Heather. So, we brought her into my office and Ken sat her on my desk and said, "Heather, you made a new friend today."

"I did?" she asked.

"Yes, His name is Jesus."

"Jesus?"

"Yes, Heather. Your new friend is Jesus and He cares about you. Heather you can really have anger fits. I know because I've seen them and heard them. You know when you yell and call people names?"

"Yes," replied the strangely quiet Heather who only looked at Ken.

"Well, I want you to yell and call on the name of your new friend when you are angry, okay?" As Heather agreed, Ken had her to show him one of her angry moments. She yelled, kicked the wall and cursed. After a few minutes Ken stopped her and asked her to now yell, kick and call only on the name of her new friend, Jesus. Heather practiced and practiced yelling and hitting and kicking the wall calling out only the name of Jesus. Ken told her that was a good job and asked her to call on Jesus every time she was mad. She agreed.

"Heather, I know you have nightmares," Ken continued. He knew this because sometimes they were so difficult the staff would call me late at night and I'd come to hold Heather. Often I sang, "Jesus Loves You Heather" and prayed with her as she went back to sleep.

Heather was surprised but acknowledged, "Yes, I have bad dreams." Ken then told her that her new friend cared and he instructed her to quietly, even in a whisper, call "JESUS" when she was afraid. She agreed.

Ken then with boldness that caused me to cringe asked Heather, "Is there any other problem you have?"

Without hesitation Heather said, "I need a Mommy." Ken quickly assured her that her new friend cared about that and would help her if she asked Him. He practiced a prayer with Heather asking for a Mommy. Though I was concerned the tears on my cheek were a statement to God for help for Heather.

Remember that the reconciliation with my family was fragile? Well, my youngest sister Mary called me to tell me that she and her husband had moved from Dallas to his family's farm and that in this simpler lifestyle they were going to adopt children, older children that no one wanted. The day Charles asked me to take his children I thought of my sister with whom I spoken only a few days before.

To make a long story short, Heather practiced yelling and calling on her new friend Jesus for many weeks. It was strange hearing a 6 year old throwing a fit to Jesus. One night, about 11 p.m., I stopped by the shelter just to greet the night worker and walk through the buildings. As I neared Heather's room I heard a sound and quietly approached to learn that Heather was saying, "Oh my friend Jesus, help me. I am afraid, come to me." She was talking quietly and with a familiarity that caused me to know she was going to be okay. Through the legal avenues, after talking with my sister and hearing her desire for Heather, I gave her name as a possible placement home. My sister and her husband came to visit Heather and a younger brother, Blade. I think the placement of these children into my sister's home was done in a record time and the adoption followed in due course. A couple neat side notes to this story are that, one; I got to fly these two kids when the state placed them with my sister in Missouri. That was the initial contact with my family following the prison year and it was not about me but about the two children placed with my sister. It was a healing and special time for me. About a year later as the adoption was being finalized Heather told my sister, "I've been Heather for a long time and I am getting a new last name so I want a new first name. My new name is Margaret and you can call me Maggie." There are several awesome stories about Maggie that maybe one day she'll share, but this I know God's Spirit touched her deeply at a very young age and there is a potential in her that can only develop as she lives for God. And this too I know; she touched our family causing all of us to reconnect with God.

Leaving the shelter work was difficult for me. I had been given much respect and authority in the development of the programs for the children, and I had learned how to work as a believer in God. However, it was time to move into a new work and so I resigned and took a job as an investigator with Child Protective Services.

Chapter Four: HIV Status

Ken's words

During the days of working at the shelter we spent hours in the desert. Randy, our friend from the mobile home park, showed us all the great spots to walk and he taught us a lot about this place where we lived Don, our friend from the shelter, and I spent hours walking, hunting and talking about God. He was a special friend and I miss him. Life moved us apart, and you know it is tough to be friends with Johna and me. Maybe it is because Johna and I are such good friends or maybe because we are too intense or maybe we are just too prickly; nevertheless it seems like we have a tough time keeping friends. Whatever, Don was my friend and I learned to talk freely about God with him. He is a very successful businessman and a great musician. He knew things about art, music and people that I've never considered and, in those areas, he was my teacher. We had a good trade-off because I was more involved with things of God and certainly had more experience at hunting and so became his teacher in those areas.

In the midst of these males friend I thought of Shawn. Remember, he is the guy who took me to the hospital when Johna was in prison. I told Johna that I needed to find him and so I called the People With AIDS Coalition [PACT] of Tucson. Shawn was gay. I hoped against all odds to locate him. Shawn answered the phone and he remembered me! This was the beginning of a time of volunteering at PACT. I would go there a couple times a week and move items, talk with people, read from the Bible, and hang out. It was neat how accepted I was and that is probably because of Shawn. He educated me about the gay lifestyle telling me stories of his experiences in the bath houses in San Francisco and he helped me understand his perception of the why and what of being homosexual. I really liked Shawn.

Shawn told me the following pieces of his story as he explained his position on God, homosexuality and HIV. I've included this little story as a way of sharing his perceptions with you.

"Just what is a man's place?" Shawn thought. How long had he been uncertain? Two years? Three? Maybe more. Anyway, he was 14 years old now and he sure as hell didn't know the "man's place in life". The 14-year-old boy shuddered and zipped his light jacket the rest of the way up. He lowered his head and walked across the street to the bar door and hesitated only briefly before entering. Twenty minutes later he left with a man thirty years his senior. They went to what was, in those days, called a 'bathhouse.' The boy's life was forever changed. It was much later in his life, of course, that I came to know Shawn. He'd been openly gay for several years and at the time was in the business of, what else, hair cutting. He was 36 years old and already knew of his HIV+ status. In fact, Shawn was the first homosexual I ever really knew and he was the first person with AIDS with whom I was privileged to become friends. I don't think we were the usual

friend either of us was accustomed to having, but for me it was valuable relationship. I would sit and listen to stories about his gay lifestyle and was sickened in my spirit. The levels of decadence and the unceasing appetite for even more shocked and annoyed me. Some of his stories were so bizarre I doubted they were true but he told them in vivid detail and I always thought he was working to shock me into removing myself from any exchanges with him.

I looked a bit in the library about the role of the San Francisco ill-famed bathhouses as to the spread of AIDS in this country, but I did not read of such things as Shawn described to me. He talked about boys, 14 years old and younger, taken to these large, he said 300 room, facilities with open pools, hot tubs and saunas and being literally passed around by the older men. Shawn told of a 12 hour, seven-dollar pass that enabled him to gain unescorted entry into such a place. He claimed to have spent many hours in those bathhouses.

During the time in the bathhouses he might have sex with 30 or 40 different men, most of whom he did not know. Now Shawn was not paid to do this, at least not most of the time. He was not a prostitute in the sense of the word of getting paid for sex or having sex with others as a job. He was a lonely 14-year-old boy who felt he could not satisfy his family and primarily his father. He talked of his dad as a military man of some rank who rarely was home. Shawn described with pride his father's military achievement and we all knew he loved his dad. Yet the two were nothing alike. I once asked Shawn, "What is it about men that appeal to you?"

"That's simple. I love their strength. With a strong man I feel safe."

I thought that was so odd because Shawn was slightly built but not petite and not feminine. I wondered what scared him so? What was the fear that caused him to so need to feel safe? I have yet to understand.

Shawn and I talked about God, Jesus and spiritual things, and I found him well versed about religion, in fact fundamental religious belief, but far from a belief that God is or that God cared about Shawn. I was curious about his past but we never really talked too much about it, he was very careful to guard his family. In fact, he told me that Shawn was a name he chose and paid for in court.

I knew Shawn for about three years. I was told today he died. It seems the disease that normally takes it time to kill a person has the potential to destroy a life suddenly. Shawn died with cardiac arrest and without warning. I sat with the phone in my hand, stunned. It is hard to believe. I wish Shawn had heard me speak of God in a way that would have helped him. He was so defiant and it seemed like his choices came from a place in his emotions that drove him. Even knowing he was HIV+ he continued having unprotected sex. Shawn's choices came out of his need and left him always needing more.

"Hey Ken, Preacher Boy, you ought to get a HIV test. You know you come here and are helpful and that is part of your job, but my job is to get people to test for HIV. I bet you have not always been such a Preacher Boy, huh?" Shawn was challenging me again and I wanted to respond appropriately in God's eyes.

"You are right Shawn. I've shot drugs and had sex with more than a few women. I will test." So, they drew some vials of blood from my arm and gave me a number along with some literature and an encouragement to return in two weeks. The card had the date and time written on it. I assured them I'd be back. Once home I read the literature and sat down feeling a strong sense of dread. I called Johna.

Johna's words

Ken has been volunteering at PACT. I'm not sure what this is about. The other day he told me, "The guys are nice. They let me in to help but I need a passkey. Johna, if ever I will make a difference with this group something has to change. I never thought homosexual guys would be a place assigned to me for speaking Jesus. But, you know Johna; they have taught me a lot. If we as Christians cared as much about one another as gay guys care about their friends we'd made a huge difference in our communities." Ken called me at work asking me to come home. He sounded weird so I arranged time off and left.

"Ken I'm home." Where was he? I heard a sound and found him in the restroom. Our Airedale, Malchus, was the clue as he sat against the bathroom door whining. "Ken, are you okay?"

He emerged from the restroom. He was pale and directly came and hugged me saying, "Here, sit here and let's talk." Ken then told me about Shawn's challenge and handed me the literature. Actually, it was one piece of literature that Ken had marked what he wanted me to read. The handout talked about HIV and listed ten early warning signs. As I read the list I knew. Ken had marked his symptoms and I knew. In truth neither of us knew that much about HIV but we were not stupid. HIV meant AIDS and that meant death. We knew that Ken was HIV positive. I looked at Ken and he said, "Oh Johna what have I done to us?" We held each other and were quiet. I called to work the next day asking for a sick day.

Ken shares

I didn't want to go get the test results but never seriously considered not going. We learned that 40% of people tested do not return to learn the results of their test. It is, I guess, too hard. Johna and I dressed up and she took the day off so we could go hear the results at 10 a.m. and then have some time to "process the fact" whatever that might be.

My friends were not in the lobby that day when Johna and I entered the PACT facility. The clinic felt strange and concerning. I was not treated like a volunteer but like a client. The wait was brief and then Johna and I were in the room with a woman who talked and talked. Finally she gave me a paper and told me that three tests are done to determine if person is HIV+ and that the tests are 99.99% accurate. All three tests showed that I was HIV+ and, by the way, Johna must be tested. And, oh by the way, I'd get better services if Johna and I divorced and hey you need to know, I was told, that you will live about another four years. It was 1992 when I tested HIV positive. I had the passkey into the land of people with HIV/AIDS. I wondered what it would open.

Johna's words

Shut up! I wanted the person at PACT to just shut up. We didn't know enough about HIV to even have an opinion and they were telling us to divorce, that Ken was going to die in a few years and that I must be tested now. Okay, I gave blood and then told Ken we needed to leave. He agreed. We went home and for the next three weeks you know what we did? We ate, I worked as few hours as possible and we wrapped ourselves in blankets even though it was July 1992 and we watched old movies. Oh, and at week two we went back to PACT where we learned that I tested HIV negative, but hey that doesn't mean much and I needed to test again in about four months and Ken had to have some other testing done. Shawn was very helpful and scheduled it and had Ryan White money, because Ken wasn't on my insurance due to lack of our money, pay for it. We had an appointment in another couple weeks.

Soon after we learned that Ken was HIV+ there was an experience that caused me to love God different. It was as if I was placed, again, on the balance beam and I knew that I knew a choice was given me. It was okay if I decided to not be part of the HIV situation. I could leave and God would love me, protect me and help me. However, if I stayed the choice had to be one of forever because there were things associated with Ken's HIV status that could only be known as we lived with it. Again, I was careful. To my mind came the remembrance that choosing Ken was agreeing to great love, great pain, and great everything and here, sure enough, was a great disease. His grace, the Bible tells us, is sufficient and I knew there was no way this situation could be carried except in Christ Jesus. Ken is my great love and there was no need for deliberation. My response was yes and amen, so be it. In that moment, though I didn't realize it, my life changed again.

Ken was so quiet these days. Malchus, our dog, was his constant companion. It came to me that Ken needed a bull terrier and so I looked and found one in California. Belle, as Ken named her, was too expensive but she has, these 11 years but worth every penny. There is no better dog. As time went by I learned from Belle, Katie Belle we often call her, when Ken is having a "bout with the HIV". Really. Belle will stay very close to Ken, lick his limbs and whine a few days before he is sick, and

I've learned that the smell of HIV will be strong in Ken a few days after Katie's display of concern. We love her and she is old and we pray for her often. Don loaned us his sports car and we drove, fast, across the state to meet the owners and pay the money to have Belle.

Belle broke the feeling of sadness and despair from us. A puppy in the house was fun. Malchus was only kind and accepting of her. There will not be a dog as kind as Malchus. We named him for the guard that had his ear cut off by Peter and replaced by Jesus. Malchus had an ear that drooped. He died too young of cancer and we buried him on the property west of town and thinking about him makes me sad. He was a good dog. Ken taught him to "gun fight." Ken would say, "Malchus, there is not enough room in town for the two of us." Malchus would crouch down and sneak up toward Ken then running the last few yards for a greeting and hugs. It was very cute.

After the trip to get Belle we told Don and Nancy, our friends and she was my supervisor at the shelter, about Ken's HIV status. They sat a model for the work we do with HIV positive people. They didn't realize the impact, perhaps, on us but it was strong. We were brought into sanctuary. Their concern and love was without condition and it was strong. Sanctuary means a place where agents stand against the forces that cause the harm. Don and Nancy were sanctuary for us. They stood against us eating barely enough, they stood against us being without a car, and they were always encouraging us in faith that God is big enough for all the situations of life. And, they did this without judgment. We thank them and we work to provide such a place for the friends we know who are HIV infected or affected.

One of many things Don and Nancy did for us was provide, in about January after learning of Ken's HIV+ status, a cabin at Pine Top. At that place we could talk about what HIV+ meant and by that time we had researched it a lot. We cried and loved one another and prayed and we were better when we returned from this vacation. In fact, Ken decided that telling his family was important. His sister, Karla's death, influenced him and the comments made by his parents of "I wish" and "If only". So, we called Harold and his wife Lois and it was a good thing that Lois, in her job, had just had a in-service about HIV/AIDS. Then we called Ken's mother, Barb and her husband, Max, and talked with them. It wasn't long after that that they visited us.

One really pleasant memory was the trip with Max and Barb to Orlando. We toured NASA, ate fish and messed with alligators, enjoyed Disney World and the other attractions and became acquainted with

Max and Barb. Back then; everyone thought Ken would die in a year or two. That's what the doctors told us. I remember his T-Cell count was about 700 and that was pretty good. A healthy person will have a T-Cell count of 1200 to 1500 per little bit of blood so Ken was doing okay but we watched him carefully.

In fact, I wore myself and him out keeping track of what he ate, how much he slept and voided and etc. etc. We both were relieved when I gave that kind of attention up!

Ken shares

I will always thank the Lord for Cindyrae and Andy who initiated my first contact with Hampton. They have listened to God's directions many times, and in their obedience others benefit. It was March 3rd and a beautiful day, the first good sun in weeks. I was wandering the yard appreciating the glory all around me; too many shades of green to number, early wild flowers in brilliant bloom, sky so blue painters dare not copy it. I am thankful. I'm thankful that I am aware of God. His presence lifts me and I see a deeper layer than I otherwise am capable of knowing. God has said His ways are not our ways. His ways are higher than ours. There are days when shame threatens to consume my thoughts and when I must fight to even leave the house. I had lots of shame for my condition, yes, but more because I realize the advantages that I wasted. My shame is that it took this, AIDS, before I cared enough to try to make a difference. As immobilizing as shame can be yielding it to Christ is completely liberating! I miss Hampton.

When I first spoke with Hampton he was working evenings, I think, at the hotel. We were both nervous not knowing anything about each other except that we shared AIDS. I'm not sure if Hampton knew anyone else with AIDS at the time but I did not. Everyone I had known from PACT had already died. Hampton and I visited for about 10 minutes I guess but I sensed we had made some sort of connection. Hampton was always so easy to talk with and he was a wealth of information about this disease.

I think the next time we spoke Hampton had just been fired or let go or whatever they called it. He was pretty down and if I remember right his latest counts weren't that great either. Even so, we laughed about things because Hampton could always see a humorous side. I admit that as I dealt with my early awareness of my own HIV/AIDS it was

Hampton's positive outlook that encouraged me and helped lend hope. I miss that.

I just looked up and the *Price Is Right* in on TV. We watched it one of Hampton's last good days at the hospital. I think he would have made a wonderful teacher. He was thorough, patient and always well researched. Hampton's varied interests often surprised me. When we talked about Jesus his innocence and purity would captivate me. The Lord calls for us and says we must approach Him as a child, but I never really saw it before seeing it in Hampton. He trusted and believed without a thought of being betrayed or disappointed. He was pure of heart. I knew the voice of the Tender, the Shepherd, our Lord and I know that voice was tender toward Hampton. I felt the Lord when I was with Hampton. There was His peace.

On days like today when I am thinking about Hampton and missing him most, he has been dead some years now, I picture him in heaven, wide-eyed taking everything in. I picture him robust, happy, with a smile that's, well, a Hampton smile. I see him in a glorious white tunic with a gold belt and a flowing turquoise robe. I still see him bald and maybe that is because I liked that look on him. Thinking about heaven makes you long to be there and if I have a vote about where my home is located I want it near Hampton's.

Johna's words

I am grateful for this person named Hampton. Ken talks with him a lot and it helps. They talk about the medication and Hampton has been on about all of it. We don't know much about his life, but he is our friend. I wonder whether there will be a time when we are involved with people living with AIDS. I think about the day we were encouraged to "get a divorce so you'll get more services." What's up with that kind of thinking? We have a lot to learn. Ken encourages me to see the hurtful statements of people as an opportunity to educate that means we must become more knowledgeable about this disease and its impact on others.

It is weird to tell my family about Ken but I need to because this fact is so big in our life that it colors everything else. However, what can they think but that I'm on another con? They have already experienced one illness lie. Valerie and Mary were both were kind and gentle with me as I told them about Ken's HIV+ status. It is good to talk with them and I'm glad they know. Eventually I told or had my younger sisters tell all the people in my family about Ken's status. Not many of them really know him and in fact I don't know my family. Mother, Valerie and Mary know me. We have all changed so much and it takes time and exchanges to build back trust. There hasn't been opportunity for that with most of my family.

AIDS is consuming and Ken and I know that we must get involved and I think and he is okay with the idea that we educate the Church. Even in our own church we've heard statements like, "When all the drug addicts and gays are dead there won't be a problem." That is not true and the prejudice is painful. We set up an appointment, in 1995, and talked with the pastor and his wife about Ken's status and the growing need in us to be a voice of education. They were very supportive and encouraging. We provided some education at our church and then, from various contacts, we were educating in a lot of different churches. Most of the churches were very conservation and they were both large and very small in number. We developed a quick way of helping a church create policies and procedures and then to institute universal precautions. It was not difficult. I am amazed at how we, the Church, say we are the safe place for all hurting people and yet a disease causes so many political and social problems even in the small congregations. I became bold reminding the leaders that it is likely that HIV+ people already attend their church and unless there is education there is risk. One time I asked the pastor's wife whom I knew had grandchildren, "Do your grandchildren stay in the nursery?" When she affirmed they used the nursery I asked her, "And what precautions are being practiced there that cause you to feel safe for your grandchildren?" We did a lot of work with that church.

Ken's point of view

Johna and I need to do something about HIV/AIDS. We talk about it all the time. She is ready to give up her work in the prisons and has found another woman to whom the responsibility of Prison Fellowship will be transferred. That has been a marvelous time for us but it has ended. She has one more time of speaking in a church about recruiting women to volunteer in the prison and then her commitments will end. I feel like we are going into a land of famine and AIDS is the wagon on which we can take the Bread, the good news of Jesus. I am not sure if the land of famine is the Church or the people living with AIDS.

Our pastor set up a dinner with some people from the church who have money and were interested in giving some to a ministry to people with AIDS. The pastor could not attend the dinner and we felt nervous. We talked about what and how much to say. We decided that we'd respond to the questions. We had not been served the food when our dear friend Walt asked, "Tell us about you." Well, Ken and I looked at one another and in about two sentences said it all and that can be summed up by, "Ken worked many years on the railroad, got involved in drugs and met Johna at a drug rehab center where she was hiding out trying to commit suicide because she didn't want to face the music of going to prison. And, yes Johna did go to prison and now we are trying to deal with the fact that Ken has HIV."

That's a lot to lay on a couple wanting perhaps less and desiring to give money to help ministry to people with AIDS. But you know we felt they ought to know to whom they might entrust their money. Walt and Jill gave money and in May 1996 a not for profit organization called Casa Gloriosa was established with the mission of being sanctuary to people who are HIV infected or affected or who are living with AIDS. Not only did they give and continue to give money, they gave support to the agency and to us. They remain our dear friends.

It was early and we seemed to have beaten the crowd. The clinic is always busy, always filled with folks representing various maladies and afflictions. It's very sad, the number of ill, I mean we live in an age of technology and the application of science and medicine change continual to improve the human condition. And yet so many are sick, hurt and downtrodden. "Ken Reeves!" my turn had arrived and I entered the small sterile room to have blood drawn yet again. The doctors take blood to monitor my condition. They run tests and are very interested in the T Cell Count. You see, it cannot be known how a person is just by looking. The person may look healthy on the outside while on the inside things are going on that should not be. So too, the spiritual condition is not always visible, easily seen or correctly diagnosed. "Ken?" My nurse, a woman of 50 something politely calls me back and I lay out my arm so the needle can be inserted. I've been doing this for more than 4 years now and know some of the clinic staff but I didn't know this lady. I watched as she put on the thin latex gloves that were her protection from accidental exposure to HIV. Not much of a barrier when you're dealing with life or death. I wondered if she thought the same.

The nurse filled 7 vials, one about the size of my thumb and six the size of my little finger. I have big hands.

When the nurse finished I said, "You left me some?"

She smiled and answered, "A little bit."

"It's no good anyway," I added with a chuckle. As I said, I didn't know this nurse, didn't know her name or anything about her but when her eyes met mine, in that moment of my casual remark, I knew one thing, she was a mother. Quickly I said, "But, it's better than none."

The nurse smiled, "Yes," she said, "It's better than none."

In a few weeks my physician will know how I'm doing and whether the virus has advanced and if my immune system had weakened. But, the true test of my condition isn't told in a blood test and can't be determined in a lab. The Great Physician knows my heart, His Word is my medication and His diagnosis is exact. I give my blood to the clinic but my faith is in Jesus Christ.

There was an article about a drug being used that I'd never heard of it so I reached for the phone. On the second ring Hampton picks up and I am instantly warmed at his soft hello. It's a good day he says though I'm not sure how much discomfort his definition allows. I'm sure as I ask my questions that Hampton can sense my anxiety. He rarely shows his; however, and he calmly fills me in on the medicine. I have a consultation with the doctor and I am pretty sure she'll talk with me about the medication. Johna too believes that there will be a presentation requesting I start the antiviral medications. As I write this I am sad. Hampton, I miss him. Yes it's mostly for selfish reasons. He calmed me. He helped me understand the medical position of dealing with AIDS. Part of my decision regarding the drug therapy is based on his frankness and openness with me.

Johna shares

I went with Ken to his doctor's appointment today. His T-Cell count is still strong. The doctor wants him to consider taking the HIV medications and she has offered to set up a consultation with the leading HIV doctor in town. I listen as Ken tells her he isn't ready to take medication. We then talk about the progression of this disease and I leave the office heavyhearted knowing that this is an issue we will have to face sooner or later.

Ken's words

In July 1996 our church had a family camp over the Fourth of July weekend and a person from South Africa was brought in as the speaker. In the Pentecostal milieu he is known as a Prophet. Johna and I attended these services, sat on the side of the building and tried to not bring attention to us. Ron Campbell, special speaker, asked us to come up on the platform at the front of the church. The following is the word he spoke to us:

> God says I've placed you in this place and I'm going to start using you in a great anointing. You have an understanding of the things of God. I've taken you out of lost place and brought you to a found place At one stage you were rejected as a son but I am raising you up to be a Father and you'll be a father to the lost and unwanted. He is causing life to come into body and bones, both of you. Your days of struggling financially are over. There are those that have despised and spoken against you. Rebuke the devourer on your behalf. I'm opening doors of opportunity and there is even promotion in the Spirit. Where in the past you've been overlooked you are now going to be used and blessed. This blessing is seed, it is seed not to be eaten but it is seed to be planted. God says, I see you preparing places. Places for people to stay, people who are hurt and lost. You have heart for young women who have been broken through rape and rejection and illegitimacy you are going to become a love mother to them. I'm releasing anointing on you right now. You'll bring them into the Kingdom raise up many dancers, worshippers and musicians. I am releasing the anointing of restoration, right now. This time will prepare you to move about the city and even the nation. But for now your season is in the house and it is the season to be hidden. There will be a time for exile to be released and you will move around the nation. God, bless this couple.

In the same time frame of Ron Campbell visiting our church Johna was invited to attend another church where the pastor John Aker was very supportive of Prison Fellowship. He was going to give her a few minutes, in the middle of his sermon, to speak about the need for volunteers for the work of Prison Fellowship. We were excited to speak and this was the last engagement Johna had before the newly appointed woman would take over this volunteer work. We had talked with John Aker previously and shared my HIV status and the fact that we were going to initiate a work with people who were living with HIV/AIDS. In the break between the services Pastor Aker spoke with us saying that he thought it would be a good opportunity for us to share about Casa Gloriosa and the work with HIV people; however he felt that would require us to disclose my HIV status. I immediately agreed with him. Johna then asked, after the Pastor left us, if I planned to come up to the front with her. Of course not! It was her speaking engagement and I believed it would be more effective if I did not come to the front with her.

Johna shares

Here I was in front of more than 1000 people and I didn't know more that maybe 10 of them and I disclosed that my husband was HIV+. It happened so fast or I might not have been able to share that fact. At that point we had told several people but I had personally told only a person or two and then 1000. I knew that day was a marker in the work of Casa Gloriosa. The church people seemed to absorb the fact and my hurt. I was glad that Pastor Aker had made space for us. When we arrived home there were 17 phone calls and most were people who hurt because of HIV/AIDS being in their life and the ones that caused me to cry were the old mother's of adult children who were homosexual and/or with AIDS and these mothers were thanking us for sharing about the disease and Ken's status. I knew we were launched into the work of caring about people with HIV/AIDS.

We were in a short time invited to speak to a group of people at this same church, Christ Community Church. We talked to a small group and one woman caught my heart. Sharon. We learned, a little later, that she was Hampton's mother. It is a small world. Sharon caused me, by her pain and her determination to be what her son needed, to be resolved to do this work. In the course of a short time she then introduced us to a friend who had a property for sale. The Christian community, especially Grace Chapel, encouraged us to buy a property and serve women with HIV/AIDS. Women were the target we felt needed service and there was nothing designed especially to meet their needs. So, we looked at the property and knew it was an answer.

Ken shares

Johna and I went to the property. It was in good shape, a triplex converted into an adult care home and the sweet old people living there were going to have to move because the managers could no longer continue the work. The house had eight bedrooms, five bathrooms, two common areas, and a kitchen and laundry facility. Because of Sharon's influence the owner was prepared to give us a very good deal. We talked with the pastor of our church and he felt the church could raise the down payment and would pay the monthly mortgage until the agency was established.

Johna's words

In the process of deciding to buy the property for a shelter for people with HIV/AID we visited a home for people with AIDS located in Washington State. The Christian community there supported it and the work was good. This was a great visit for me and we made some lifelong friends. One observation that I consider often is the lack of prayer covering that work. I knew that we must have strong prayer people and we set out to make certain that, in the midst of doing good deeds, we didn't neglect the true work of any effort for God, prayer. Some of our friends immediately started praying about the property and it was a regular event to have between 3 and 10 people go to the location and pray that God would work on behalf of the people with AIDS and Casa Gloriosa to give the building to this work.

In November of 1996 we rented the facility on Bryant Street calling it GLORY HOUSE. So many people came and worked and cleaned and fixed up. Dad Casteel who became and remains the chaplain of the agency was in his eighties but he has worked and worked and worked on behalf of people with HIV/AIDS. His influence toward us has been significant. One time I shared with him my feeling of tiredness and he told me, "Johna, go for the deep water. When you get in the middle of it a horse will come and carry you. Now you weary yourself splashing in the shallow water." I'll never forget that and am always encouraged to head on out into the deep water of obedience to the call of God. In 2000 Dad and his wife Louise visited Ken and me at Glory House and his words that day have been part of the sustaining force during these days when Ken has been so ill. He told us, three times, that day that we had unusual faith. Now Dad Casteel is not a man to flatter or praise. He speaks as he believes and sees it and he has lived faithful to God many years. His words came at a time when we did not receive them with pride or arrogance but knew that God who had started the good work in us is faithful to continue it and we bowed before Him again confessing our willingness to be willing.

Another person who gave many hours and hard work was a Registered Nurse and she took it on herself to clean the bathrooms. I've used her work as a model many times in the orientation of volunteers. She did not expect special treatment because of her position as a RN but rather she humbled herself and did a very good job of making sure the toilets, sinks and tubs were ready to serve people. And, you know, she did the labor with a smile and a song in her heart and mouth. She was the first to bring her children into the house of AIDS. I love the picture of her and her daughter painting cabinet doors!

The Glory House facility was purchased with money raised from the church in January 1997. In November of 1996 we rented the building and right away two people moved into it. A man and his four-year-old son who was HIV+ moved into the building for a month. He agreed to clean and paint a couple of rooms in exchange for staying in the facility. This man left in a few weeks and I later heard his son had died. The other young man was a friend of Hampton, Bobby, and he needed a place to stay.

We really liked having Bobby in the house. He was good at cleaning and making people who came to clean or repair the facility feel welcome. He stayed with us a couple different times and remains one of our friends who will always have a place in our heart and home. We had an open house early in 1997 and were ready for women to admit and no one came. Ken and I looked at each other and quietly waited. It was one of those times Ken encouraged my faith by telling me, "This is God's work and He will bring the people as well as pay the bills. If we've missed it we might as well know right now!"

The day the offering was taken at the church a young girl, maybe 11 years old, gave 53 cents and she continued to give a monthly sum with her largest gift reaching $5.

When I would feel overwhelmed by the work we were entering I'd think about that sweet gift and recall the angels of the children who come day by day before God's face. From the beginning of this work the model was to provide sanctuary. Remember, to me sanctuary is a place of safety and belongingness that is created by agents that stand, tall and strong shoulder to shoulder, against the forces that would hurt, destroy and kill. It is my firm belief that the most appropriate and the fiercest agents for the community of people living with HIV/AIDS are people of faith. Ken and I wanted a place where infected and affected people felt treasured, protected and where truth prevailed

Ken shares

The media came during those first days of Casa Gloriosa. One of the reporters interviewed me and without thinking I responded to a question with, "This is an answer to prayers not yet prayed." In the years since we started that response has been true over and over. As the children come into the programs and the Glory House I realize that God started us in a direction we could not have considered in the smallness of our minds and heart. He has taken us into a place bigger than I would have been willing to go had I known. And then I think of the beginning of this journey that started with a prayer, "Oh God, if you are show me and I am willing to be willing to know you completely."

I might have been able to answer, in part, that Glory House was an answer to prayers not prayed because I'd written a little story. This story fits some of the children we have come to love who are HIV positive and so I'll share it with you.

Every morning when dawn's faintest stroke would brush the black night away, her eyes would flutter open. She would smile almost sheepishly and say, "I'm still alive!"

Cassandra's indomitable spirit captured us all. Her mother was full blown AIDS at the time of delivering Cassandra into this world. Her father was a street junkie who was also HIV+ and would never even know of his daughter's existence. "I'm still alive!"

Cassandra was five when she first came to Glory House. Doctors continued to be amazed at her endurance and spoke of her "will to live" as perhaps her greatest asset. Cassandra disagreed. She knew it was Jesus. She used to tell us, "I don't know why I want to live so badly, but I do."

Cassandra knew, that is she understood about Christ, about His laying down His life her, about His rising again and about Jesus in heaven now awaiting her. Still she said, "I know Jesus will take me when I'm ready but I keep saying just a little longer Jesus, just a little longer." And then she'd giggle as if she were really being spoiled. Cassandra didn't feel as if she had a great mission to attend or anything like that, but she realized that heaven would be forever and Cassandra truly loved life. Isn't that pitiful? I mean all she ever really knew was heartache, hardship and suffering and yet Cassandra hung on fiercely fighting overwhelming odds. I remember the day Cassandra turned seven. She had been quite ill for several months and barring an actual miracle Cassandra would not see eight. I look forward to the day when I see Cassandra in heaven.

Chapter Five: Casa Gloriosa

Johna's point of view

In April the women begin to fill the house. At this point we did not have a manager in the home believing that the adults could take care of themselves with the little bit of overseeing I could provide. During all these early years, from 1996 until mid-2001, I worked a full time job and Ken and I were volunteers with the agency. Actually from April 1997 until about June 2000 63 people lived at Glory House. The occupancy permits allows only 12 people to reside there at a given time. The average length of stay was 4 months with some staying almost two years. The women taught us and Ken and I were at the house as much as we could because the learning curve for us was interesting and exciting and these first women were our teachers.

My job at Child Protective Services was also providing valuable lessons. I worked as an investigator in the night unit. This unit had the best supervisor in the county, and I think probably the state, so all the workers were really good and all of them had a heart for the children. We became a tight knit group and much of my support, in terms of balancing a husband with HIV, working full time and trying to establish an agency, came from this group. They were interested in the response of the church and were truthful in the feedback they'd give me. Personally I owe a lot to this group of people. Some of the cases assigned to me were very difficult and we worked 10 hours for eight evenings plus some all nights as the on call person, and then we were off 6 days. These hours allowed me time to do the work for Casa Gloriosa but there were days in a row when Ken and I hardly saw one another. In some of those early morning CPS calls, that might take me to a hospital or to a police scene, I would find myself calling on God to bring energy, clarity of thought and assistance. On time I was on the way home, maybe 3 a.m., after seeing a child with badly burned hands, that the Spirit of God really touched me. The mother held her son's hands over an open gas flame because she wanted to teach her four year old mildly retarded son to not play with the stove. I'll never forget the look in that child's eyes. I so wanted to help him. There was no one in the emergency room with him and I stayed hours. At one point he laid his head on my arm. I prayed, out loud, for this little boy I'll call Joey.

Driving the 18 miles home I sobbed, emotionally, spiritually and physically undone. As I looked to heaven for help I thought again of the angels of the children and I recalled that we have both angels and ministering spirits assigned to us. I asked for help and immediately felt the warm touch of the Spirit of God deep inside me. You may think this weird but until you've been in the situation where a child is badly hurt and see his/her pain and are limited in what you can do, don't be so cynical. God loves the children. After sleeping a few hours Ken and I had breakfast and talked about how God wants to be involved in all we do or say, but we really fight to look, act and seem politically and socially correct and that means avoiding a direct partnership with God. I was reminded of one reason I so love Ken. He does not waver, he is a man with an opinion, he believes what he believes and living with him is always an adventure as he puts all of life under the power and authority of God.

My Mother visited and I was invited to a visit with my sisters and mother at our aunt's place in Texas. These exchanges helped all of us see another more clearly. For me seeing Mother was always good and she never failed to talk with me about "being true to what you believe God is asking of you." She told me a story one of these visits about her good friend who had been a missionary to South America for many years. When I was arrested, or in prison, Mother received a letter from this friend encouraging her to only pray for me and telling me she believed that, if I would allow God to control my life, I would have "kingdom value". I would have kingdom value, what a goal and how unbelievable! My Mother always encouraged me but she also challenged me.

Mother's influence caused me to want the clients coming to Casa Gloriosa to be embraced in the manner of Jesus. I believe this means doing and not saying Jesus, it means to refrain from requiring an organized prayer time, devotional time or a requirement of church attendance. This position caused some of the churches we visited to not support the work. In order to get some money a Bible class must be required for the clients or the church must be allowed to come into the facility for a healing or prayer service. We believe the method of touching people with HIV/AIDS is giving the kindness, the consistency and the support of Jesus and to refrain from speaking doctrine, judgment or religious requirements.

Ken shares

Johna and I talked about being Jesus and prayed God would bring opportunities our way. Carmen, a volunteer, was about 18 years old when she became a tireless young woman motivated by what? I never knew her reasons except the fact she loved Jesus. Carmen volunteered for Casa Gloriosa and for another agency in town that provided care teams for people with AIDS. One day she stopped at the Casa to speak with me. She was part of a care team for a man named Kevin who was dying and she told me, "Ken, he needs Jesus, can you come pray with him? He said its okay for you to come." So, I readily agreed not knowing what lie ahead, but hey everyone needs a chance to know Jesus so I would go.

By the time I visited Kevin we were pretty much used to seeing ravaged bodies and skinny folk, but I was not prepared for the man I saw in that hospital bed. "O dear God, is that a human, a real man?" Had I not made eye contact with this fellow I might have backed out the door and not said a word. But I focused on Carmen's obvious concern and her concern was nothing compared to God's love for this person. I entered his room ready to do my little thing and get the heck out of there. This shouldn't take but a few minutes and I would be finished. It turned out Kevin was a talker and there was no escape from this visit.

As I stepped toward Kevin's bed I again prayed, "O God, there is nothing left of him." I found out later that Kevin was over six foot tall and weighed maybe 100 pounds. He had been an equestrian braider and the room was filled with pictures and mementos from healthier and happier times.

Kevin may have been forewarned about my visit because his first words to me were, "I am a Buddhist." Okay, I didn't say it but wondered, "Where are all your Buddhist buddies now that the bottom is falling out of your life?" We talked of many things and I kind of liked him. He told me about his former profession which he really had enjoyed. It was obvious that Kevin was very ill and his body was shot but he was pretty with it mentally, at least some of the time his thinking was right on. The best description I can give of my thoughts and feelings was a Jolly Roger Flag. Kevin looked like a pile of bones with a head on top of them. The most difficult aspect of visiting Kevin was the smell. I had worked in packing plants that never smelled as bad as his room. The nurses had two large window fans going full blast not for fresh air, but to take the odor out the open windows. Everyone going in his room wore masks because of the odor and I've seen some spray a fragrant into the mask before entering the room. For the most part people came into his room, did whatever had to be done and quickly got out of there. It was as if the odor and the disease of Kevin were so strong it might cling to you.

After this visit I talked with Johna and decided I would visit Kevin again, soon. I checked in at the nurse's station and then entered Kevin's room. The odor was 10 fold stronger. I had some experience, working with my step dad a bit, around burns and had worked in packing plants so I decided to deal with the odor in a manner of respect to Kevin. I didn't wear the mask. The previous work had prepared me so I was able to visit him without succumbing to the smell or the urge to get out of there. Kevin noticed the lack of a mask and I know he was pleased. Once he asked me, "Is that awful smell me?" Johna and I had agreed to truthful statements with any HIV infected/ affected person we had the opportunity to know and speak with, so I told him that yes the sores on his spine were rotting and the smell was from them. He looked me in the eyes and said, "Thanks for speaking the truth."

Johna shares

Ken had visited Kevin a couple or three times and invited me to go with him. I agreed with some reluctance knowing this would be an up close and personal contact with a person dying of AIDS. It seemed like that condition was far from us and I liked it that way. However, I went to be supportive of Ken. Ken warned me about the smell, the condition and the fact that Kevin probably would not be responsive toward me. The smell was in the hallway of the hospice, the nurses were very nice and one helped me gear up with mask, gloves and gown. Once in the room I didn't want to open my mouth the horrible smell was so pervasive. Ken introduced me but Kevin immediately started talking with Ken about his pain and I left the room fairly quickly sitting in an outside patio area fighting tears. "God whatever our journey, please protect Ken from this kind of ending." I thought about how difficult this must be for Ken and yet how unaffected he presented to Kevin except for his concern and friendship toward Kevin. I fell one more time in deep love for my husband.

Ken's words

I went to see Kevin knowing that his days were short and he had been in my prayers and thought during the night. He was agitated and told me about the bad dream that had kept him awake too much during the night. He told me, "I was being led toward a door, it was closed. When they got me to the door and tried to open it, the door wouldn't budge. They couldn't get my inside. I am scared. The door wouldn't open."

"Kevin," I replied, "That's because Buddha can't open that door. Jesus said I am the Door and Kevin He is the answer to your closed door." I remember Kevin's tears that day and was so thankful and amazed that God's grace extends to every one of us. Kevin repeated the words asking Jesus to forgive his sins and to live in his heart. In a few days Kevin died. They held his memorial in the hospital chapel.

A friend told me that the Chaplain came by later the day Ken visited and prayed with Kevin. The Chaplain had been told that Kevin was upset about a bad dream and asked Kevin if he thought God was rejecting him. Our friend told me that Kevin replied, "No, I don't believe He would reject me, not now."

I didn't want to attend Kevin's memorial but felt that it was important. There was no family in attendance but for one woman who was probably in her late 50's. I found out that she was Kevin's sister. The funeral included a time for friends and family members to share antidotes about Kevin. Time and again I thought about slipping out as the remembrances included gross sexual stories that, I'm sure, were a ploy to describe Kevin as good and political correct in his position as a gay man. After the service I approached the older woman to offer my condolences. I told her that I didn't know the Kevin about whom the stories were told and that I had become his friend only in the past few weeks.

In fact I wrote my words in a journal because of her response. I said, "Ma'am I didn't know Kevin like these. Kevin and I spent quite a bit of time together toward the end of his life and I'm sure we'll see each other again in heaven." His sister hugged me and thanked me for reaching out to her brother. She told me that she had prayed for Kevin for 20 years and that she had held out no hope for him and especially as she heard the stories about his life. Her tears, she explained, were not just because Kevin died but because she thought he had died without making peace with God.

I shared the story about the door and she and I knew God's presence. I could see this heartbroken sister respond as God's Spirit sort of sweep over her heart and then her face, her countenance changed and she was at peace. On the drive home I wept for Kevin but more for his sister. I was again brought into that place of quietness amazed at God's grace and kindness. Kevin was an example of God's never failing faithfulness and love and how God will fight for us.

Johna's words

Rene, sweet Rene, came to Glory House. By this time we had hired Leigh Anne to work with children. We had one child admitted into the facility and somehow I knew we must initiate a program for children. Hiring Leigh Anne was one of the smartest moves we ever made. She learned to hear and speak the voice of the HIV infected and affected children. Her influence continues to form the programs we have for children and youth. Rene's mother is a Christian and she needed her daughter to be in Tucson. Rene was paralyzed on one side, very involved with AIDS and needed 24 hour support seven days a week. We didn't have a manager living at the facility and the 4 or 5 other adult women residing there were self-sufficient. The chores were divided up and routine was checked a few times every day by me and/or Leigh Anne. We were not equipped to provide care for Rene; however, her mother's request moved me. I talked with Leigh Anne and she was, always, willing to take shifts caring for Rene.

Ken's words

I called her "Sis". She was only with us a month. She would brighten up with I called her sis and we all enjoyed her smile. It was my thought that she needed a bell to ring so we could respond to her needs. We still have the bell. She touched Johna deeply.

Johna's words

We stayed, her mother, Leigh Anne or myself, with Rene all the time. She was funny, beautiful and wanted to see her husband. She married a man knowing he had AIDS. She became infected and died six years later of AIDS. He came and they had a time of forgiveness, which I don't know the eternal impact on him, for Rene brought freedom. One night I was sleeping in the living room at Glory House that was just a few steps from her bedroom. The sound awakened me. It was different. I got up to explore from where it came and as I stepped in the hallway I realized it was from Rene's room.

"Rene," I spoke softly wondering who had put on music. She was propped on her side and we had eye contact and she smiled. I checked the CD player, the radio and the tape player. The music, I can only say, was clear and precise.

"Johna," Rene spoke into my ear as I leaned close to her. "It is the music of heaven. Stay with me." I thought Rene might die that night and I sat, holding her hand, once in a while moving her position and we cried as the music filled the space of her room and deep into my spirit.

Rene left for hospice a few days after the music experience. It was some days later that I visited her at the hospice and then a couple of days before she died I went to see her again. She was very much out of it and I leaned near her and asked, "Rene, do you hear the music?"

Rene rallied, I think for my benefit, and said, "I am in the music. It is heaven." I had tears at Rene's memorial service and yet there was birthed in me a sense of yearning that returns from time to time, to be in that sound. And you know what; I believe that Ken is sometimes, these days, living in the sound. He hears it differently. He hears the Word, the Scripture, which is so deep in his mind and spirit. When he talks about the Word, the sound I hear; however, is the sound of that precise and clear music.

Leigh Anne was hired in about September of 1997 when there was one baby in the facility, and by the summer of 1998 she was working with 27 children who were HIV infected or affected. We had little resource and looking back we didn't ask for enough. Our faith was still being built. The cost of the facility was about $5000 per month and there was only about $2400 committed on a monthly basis. Yet, every time every bill was paid and we were never late in getting the payment made. It was a tremendous faith builder. At one board meeting Ken had a stack of the bills piled on a table to make his point of God's goodness toward the work of Casa Gloriosa.

In the summer of 1998 Leigh Anne worked five days a week with the 27 children and youth providing fun activities and education about HIV. She drove her own vehicle and most often paid for the gasoline. I know that Leigh Anne and James "used up" at least two vehicles in the work of Casa Gloriosa. Sometime in that summer she brought up her desire to have an annual camp for the HIV infected/ affected kids. I will never forget the exchange with Ken about this program. "Of course, camp is a great time and these kids need a place where it is all about them and the impact of this disease on them."

So, CAMP GLORY was initiated. In 1999 Ken and I went to the Camp as Directors and on the way we cried thinking about much we put on and allowed Leigh Anne to assume. That first camp, I think of it as Leigh Anne's Camp, was great and it solidified the idea of developing programs to children who are HIV infected/ affected. In 1999 Leigh Anne was pregnant but she developed and implemented the summer program for the children and by that time there were at least 40 kids involved in the program. Christian Faith Center, a center city church very supportive of Casa Gloriosa, provided space for the summer program. I will never forget the response of the people at Christ Community Church when we presented the need for financial support for the camp. An offering was taken and there was money enough for all the children/ youth and counselors. Also, these churches provided their bus and driver to help take and return the kids from CAMP GLORY.

In the summer of 1999 one of our friends, Isabella, was dying. This woman's children were part of the program and they had pulled on me in ways different than I had ever previously experienced. We had a pager and the boys could get in touch with us any time they needed. They lived with a grandmother, in poverty and were always concerned about their mother. Their mother, Isabella, was pretty, a 20 year heroin addict and prostitute who was not compliant with the medical prescriptions that were designed to keep her living longer. I'll never forget an early page from one of the boys asking if I could take them to see their mother. When I picked them up he told me where to find her. Not only did these kids [age 8, 10 and 11] know where their mother was they knew the motel room and told me "someone might be in there with her." After taking them back home I returned to the motel room knocked on the door and found her very high having just been used by a man who was getting off her. The man hurriedly left and I basically carried her to my car taking her to St. Mary's hospital. The doctor later told me that she might well have died that night had I not found her. It became a habit of finding her either for her sons or the doctor. Sometimes she'd stay at Glory House that meant that Leigh Anne and/or I had to be around more, but she'd only stay a day or two, see her sons and then be gone. In the summer of 1999 we had an intern from Switzerland and she really loved Isabella. Often during those hot days Rahel, Ken and or I would visit in the home. One endearing visit

Ken had made homemade chicken noodle soup and Isabella, at our arrival seemed close to death. Her face and hands were blue and she was non responsive. Ken poured up a small amount of soup and tried to entice her in eating it. She suddenly sat up and ate some soup. There were no words exchanged and she laid back down apparently asleep. We visited for a while and as we readied ourselves to leave Isabella sat up and asked, "Hey, who put that soup together? It is good." She then was out of it again.

Some of the times I visited her alone I'd ask, "Isabella are you ready to die?" At first she would deny that death was near her; however, one day she asked if we'd read the Bible. I know Rahel often read a verse or two and so would Ken and me. Late in July Ken and I were visiting her and again I asked, "Isabella are you okay with God?"

She looked at Ken and said, "I need to pray."

Ken prayed a simple pray asking for forgiveness of sin and that the peace of God would fill Isabella, her children and family. She prayed each word, smiled and we sat a while that day holding her hand.

On Sunday before Camp Glory 1999 Ken and I visited her. As I leaned to kiss her good-bye knowing that we'd have a few minutes in the morning to pick up the boys she said, "Johna, God forgives everything."

I hope my hug and kiss conveyed my regard for her and that my words were comforting as I softly said, "Isabella if I don't see you again here I will look for you in heaven."

The next morning when we picked up the boys for camp Isabella was alert and hugged and kissed each of her sons telling them, "Go, have fun. I am okay." To me it seemed that she really wanted them to leave.

Camp Glory 1999 theme was, "GET BETTER." The first night at chapel Ken talked about the need for all of us to Get Better. He told the campers that, "This year we are going to work on getting better at understanding HIV, getting better at being kind to one another, and we will get better at understanding the people in our lives who are HIV infected. The kids cheered and the spirit of friendship was high as the evening ended.

The campus was quiet; Day One of Camp Glory 1999 had ended when the cell phone rang. It was Isabella's sister. Isabella had died and they were in route to pick up the boys. When about 30 minutes had passed I called the sister back to learn they were on their way and she asked me if I'd tell the boys. At this point I brought up the idea of waiting until morning but the family felt the boys should immediately know and she restated her request that I tell them. I called a meeting with Leigh

Anne and Ken and then Ken and I went to the oldest boy's area to tell her son. I'll never forget the tears and the laying on Ken as he cried. After a while he told Ken, "You know, my mom just got better." He didn't want to go with us to tell the other boys but agreed to meet us at our room in a few minutes. The group of older boys that year was really special and he wanted to talk with them. The middle and youngest boys cried and were very upset causing emotion in both their groups. Eventually the boys went to our room and I stayed a while with the groups and counselors talking, processing the fact of a mother's death.

We learned a lot from this experience. At the morning gathering the day after Isabella's death her oldest son told the group, "My Mom just GOT BETTER!" Watching these kids share the commonality of HIV in their families, their hopes and their pain brought resolve to Ken and me that we would do our best to provide more services to HIV infected and affected children.

At the memorial service for Isabella a sister prayed with Ken for relationship with Jesus. She told me that Isabella had been a big influence on her. This past year, 2001, I saw this sister and was so pleased to see her looking healthy. Her report is that she continues a life of sobriety and that Jesus Christ is the reason. Isabella touched me deeply. The Bible says that we are accepted regardless of the time in our life of coming to God through Jesus. Isabella was beautiful example of God's desire for people.

In December 1997 Luz and her daughter moved into Glory House as the residential manager. She worked a full time day job but was at the facility every night and on the weekend. The women really liked Luz and she has a large extended family and managed the crowd of people at the Casa with a good spirited sense of humor. Early in 1998 Maureen stayed a few nights at the Casa. We knew her children some before her stay and they became very involved in the summer program. Maureen died in the spring of 1998 and by August of that year her three children needed a place to stay while their dad completed a 14-month drug rehabilitation program. This was a significant change for the agency. One of these children is HIV+ and another is mildly mentally retarded and the oldest a teenager.

These children taught us a lot about caring for HIV infected and affected kids. They continue to be part of the Casa community and the HIV+ child is now an 11-year-old young man who does a lot of public speaking with Casa Gloriosa. His report is that his health is good because he takes him medication, as he ought, has good friend with whom he can share, and knows God. One of the things we learned about with this young man was HIV medication for children. Even when he was on the nasty tasting liquid medication he was consistent in taking it. He recently talked with me, again, about his mother and how she was sick most all his life. He spoke of missing out on a mother who really was "there for me". He explained how most of their life was with his mother and "that's probably because she was always so sick."

Ken shares

Carlos came to Casa Gloriosa. There are so many people who lived at Glory House, over 60 to be exact, that I'll not attempt to mention them all, but some of the ones that influenced the direction of the agency have to be talked about to explain how and why we are what we are today. I have listed the first names of all the people who lived at Glory House from 11/96 to 1/2002 in the back of the book. Carlos was one of the few men that were admitted to Glory House as a resident. Johna was the one who believed we should admit Carlos, and you know she was correct.

Carlos was a natty dresser. In fact the first Christmas he was with us I wanted to buy him a new pair of black cowboy boots. Johna encouraged me to spend as little money as possible since this would cut into our personal money for a gift to each other. So, my good friend Gary, whom we called Big Blessing, and I took Carlos boot shopping. His statement summed up the experience, "These are no good boots."

"Carlos, you don't want a new pair of boots?"

"From here? No." And Carlos who had looked at one boot just walked off.

He was right. We were in a store carrying very inexpensive shoes and the boots I was trying to interest Carlos into buying weren't really worth much. So, we went to a "real boot shop". Needless to say the gift Johna and I gave one another that Christmas was the joy on Carlos' face every time he put on his boots! A few weeks later we were at a wedding with Carlos and he noticed my boots. "Ken you can look better than you do. Those boots are no good. Why you wear those things? "

"They are all I have Carlos."

"No where are your good boots." He thought I had a new pair of black boots too but in fact Carlos was wearing the only new boots that would be bought that year.

Carlos was an intelligent man that taught himself English and made good money as an over the road long distance truck driver. He was from El Salvador and came into the United States many years ago through the desert. Most of the people on that trip died in the desert. Carlos was largely responsible for the ones who survived and one of those people was his niece, Dora.

Johna talks

I will never forget Dora's call to me. She is a wonderful fun-loving woman who called to ask if we could help with her uncle. He was in California in a nursing home dying of AIDS and she wanted him in Tucson close to her. She told me of her debt to him and of the frustrations she'd experienced in trying to move him to Tucson. So, after a couple talks we had a plan. A family member in California would fly with Carlos to Tucson. Dora would have his medical papers transferred and would become the medical power of attorney. Carlos arrived on a Sunday and I met Dora and her family at St. Mary's hospital. About 12 hours later he was admitted into the hospital where he remained one month. In this time Dora had his insurance established in Arizona and then he needed to be released. Well, in the month Carlos lived in the hospital Ken, Dad Casteel and I visited him. He was a love. So, I agreed and we admitted Carlos to Glory House where he changed our lives.

Ken shares

My dad, Harold, visited and these two wonderful men [Carlos and Harold] were sitting in the living at Glory House. Carlos asked Dad, at the time of his arrival, if he wanted a cup of coffee. Dad was pleased to have a cup and Carlos loved to serve. After a little time of talk Carlos asked Dad to have a cup of coffee.

"Oh no thanks, Carlos."

Carlos left the room and I followed him to hear his mumbles, "Man comes to my house and he won't have coffee with me. What's the matter with him?" Carlos could not hold on to a thought for more than a few minutes and I think Carlos drank a lot of coffee in those days. Johna and I were pleased that he saw Glory House as his home. Luz and her family were very kind and included him in all their family events.

Carlos brought a lot of pleasure to the Casa. People, after they got to know him, would drop by the house just to see Carlos. The residents, all women with HIV or AIDS enjoyed and protected him. One of my fond recollections of Carlos is arriving at the house to hear him walking through it praying in Spanish. Every time he saw Johna or me he'd thank us for our friendship and tell us that he was praying for us. One Christmas Carlos and Luz sang a song at a program, for Casa Gloriosa clients, held at Christian Faith Center. Beautiful!

We don't know how many years Carlos smoked, but he was good at it and he really enjoyed the cigarette. His physician wanted him to stop or at least slow down but Carlos would forget that he'd just had one. He would have chain smoked had we not put some limits on it. Well, what a challenge. I think Rosaline was the best because she was firm with him but would distract him to help her in the kitchen or with a cleaning task. I however, in those days spent some time with him at Glory House and developed a game Carlos came to love. I'd hid the cigarettes and he could have one when he found it. So, when he'd ask for a smoke I'd simply remind him of the game and it would generally take up to 15 or 20 minutes for him to find the cigarette. I'd put one on top of picture frame or one behind a book and he would walk about the house, it seemed on his tiptoes, looking for a cigarette. We had lots of laughter and in those days Carlos would tell me about his life in El Salvador. We became good friends. On time he told me that in the last couple years he drove cross county, he'd stop for lunch and come out and not know which way he was going or what he was driving. Carlos said, "So, I'd walk around the parking lot until I'd see, looking, looking, and I'd always see my truck. Then I'd look in the back and if there was produce I go on to Boston but anything else and I'd be on my way home, California."

Johna talks

After Carlos had been at Casa Gloriosa a couple of months he began to talk about his son. He talked of his only son and how much he loved his son and wanted him. It was our information that Carlos was not going to live long so I'd encourage the house to listen and be kind and change the subject. We had Megan, Dallas and Marge's daughter, living at Glory House and she initially primarily paid attention to Carlos. He loved her and thought she had been a truck driver with him. I think his trust toward Megan allowed him to become more honest about his distress and need to see his son. One day I came unexpectedly to Glory House to find Carlos walking the house praying in English and Spanish that "Johna find my son." When he saw me he really cried telling me God had answered his prayer and thanking me that I'd find his son, Carlitos. So, I talked with Dora and with Ken and decided that Carlos was my client and I would explore the situation. It is a long story but basically Child Protective Services became involved, and an attorney was hired for Carlos. We learned that Carlos had sole custody of his son since the child was six months old. The mother of Carlitos was found and she took her son but then didn't do what needed to happen to keep him or maintain contact with him. In fact, it was November 1998 when Carlitos was brought to Glory House to stay with Carlos. I'll never forget some of his early remarks. He would touch his dad's face saying, "You live, you live!" Evidentially he had been told that Carlos was dead. Actually this kind of statement is not that uncommon when a family is trying to deal with a member who has AIDS and that person's children. That Christmas Ken and I stayed at Glory House both Thanksgiving and Christmas with Carlos and his son. They were pleasant days and we were blessed. I called the mother of Carlitos and both Carlos and his son talked with her. I thought she might come visit, allow Carlitos to get to know her and perhaps she would be the permanent placement for him. The last contact I had with her was in January of 1999 and I made that call.

Having Carlos and his son live at Glory House was not easy. However, there were at least four other children and some adults and Luz was the manager and Leigh Anne an employee so we managed. In 1999 Carlos started really having problems with his thinking and he would walk into a walk, get lost in the house and once in a while wandered away. He had many friends and finding volunteers to spend time and supervise him was not impossible, however, some violence in his behaviors developed and he started having seizures. He seemed to know that things were not good in his health and again he hired an attorney and with Dora's assistance and many talks with Ken and me he gave us a power of attorney on Carlitos. Furthermore, Carlos made Ken and me promise that we would do all we could to see that, "My son must not go this way and that way. He must go straight and be a good man." Carlos was admitted to the hospital in July of 1999 and then placed into a nursing home where he resided until death.

Camp Glory 1999 ended and we decided that a vacation was necessary. To be honest we felt drained and uncertain of the next steps for Casa Gloriosa plus we had to make decisions about Carlos' son. We both wanted to see our families so a couple friends agreed to take over the responsibilities of Glory House and we left. Carlitos who often was called JR. left on vacation with us. My sister who had adopted Heather, who became Maggie, and her brother, had also adopted another child through our influence and we thought this might be a home for Carlos' son.

I will never forget the conversation between Ken and Carlitos or Jr. about his name. "I don't like to be called Jr.," he told Ken.

"What about Carlitos, what does that mean?" Ken asked.

"I don't know but I think it is baby something."

"Hey, how about CJ?" Ken asked. Immediately the boy's face was happy and he took the name telling and correcting us as we forget to use CJ.

Entering Missouri I heard the noise and looked in the back of the vehicle to see CJ's face pressed against the window. "What are those big things?" He was referring to trees! The trip had many such exciting discoveries. CJ could write his own chapter about being at "Grandpa Harold's" where the fishing and fun never stopped. We returned to Tucson, three weeks later, rested and resolved to continue and provide ever more services for children HIV infected and affected, and we filed for guardianship on CJ Guerra who moved into our home.

Ken shares

Angel, a young father with AIDS, touched my buddies and me deeply though I'm pretty sure he never knew that we were even in his room. I'm not sure how we came to know him, but I think his kids were part of the program and Victoria, his stepdaughter asked me to visit her dad. So, I took my group of buddies, we had Bible study a couple of times a week, and went to pray for Angel who was in hospice. These guys had expressed desire to pray for sick people. This was probably the first time of such prayer for Ricardo, a Hispanic man we dearly love who has AIDS, and Rob, my big black Christian friend. But Gary had already been part of prayer for people with AIDS and he was on the Board of Directors for the agency.

When we walked into the room only his mother was there. Angel was so thin, he was an attractive young 23-year-old man, and his mother knew he was dying. We asked to pray. Yes, his mother was waiting she told Ricardo for some men to come. Please pray. As we prayed Angel's Mother took one foot and then the other running her hands up each leg, then over his chest, both arms and touched his head and face. All the while she was quietly praying as we too prayed. It was visible love. When we finished she told us that her son was ready to die and that his soul would be with Jesus.

All my buddies were weeping plenty when we left this tender mother. It broke my heart. You know it would not have surprised me if Angel would have leaped to his feet and danced with us. In fact during the prayer his eyes opened and he looked at us seeming to know that there was prayer. If a mother's love could have caused that kind of healing response it would have happened. I will never forget Angel. His children are dear to us and we see them as often as possible. Victoria has a special place in my heart. She asked a few months after Angel's death to visit his grave and we did and once in awhile we'll review the scene when four men visited her dad and his mother in the few hours before he died.

Dad Casteel and his wife Louise, we met them at Grace Chapel years ago, and for some reason he and I became super buds. I think he saw the want to in my faith and he had been a missionary to Cuba and Mexico and he yearned to see the days when people, in the United States, would be healed as he had seen in Cuba and Mexico. We love them and still have dinner together when we can and Dad has and will always be the Chaplain of Casa. One day he was sweat running off his face working on the phones at Glory House. He even had to sit down on his rear-end because the phone lines were such a mess. There were a few of us working that day and Johna came from work to check on us and she was immediately concerned about Dad. She kept trying to get him to eat. Finally he said, "Well, I guess I need to wash my face." We knew that he was on a fast. He is an old man and he will fast and pray regularly for Casa Gloriosa, for us and for all people living with HIV/AIDS. We are blessed.

Johna shares

As all these HIV infected people came into our life, and from early in 1998 to late in 1999 we were part of 12 deaths, I came to feel like we were in one of those times where we were doing the best we could, and that is all we could do. We saw the vision but we were not there and didn't really see how Casa Gloriosa was going to fulfill it. Ken would say, "But God isn't stagnant nor is He okay with us just resting, in fact He doesn't mind us taking a beating if we learn something. What have we been asking Him for, seriously? So, now when things are tough, stand." I always think of that verse that says, "Having stood, stand." Ken reminded me that we wanted to be a standard and that Jesus was our model. Jesus, the Bible states, though he was a son he learned obedience by the things He suffered. Being a standard, according to our understanding included days and weeks and years of being obedient. We have always, even in those days we thought about quitting, known that to feel the pleasure of God on us would mean that we remained involved in the work of Casa Gloriosa. In Matthew 17 is says, "But Jesus came and touched them. Get up. Don't be afraid." There were times I could have felt afraid but I know that I know that I know that GOD IS and this is His work, not ours. So, I would recognize the BUT in life and know that Jesus always comes at those time and I would look for Him and I learned to allow His touch in those times. Then I'd listen and sure enough He always would say, "Johna get up, don't be afraid." In those words I find hope and peace and rest and strength.

And it was late in 1999 that a call from CPS was placed to me. At that time I was employed with the agency. Basically I was told that a girl had been placed, months before, from Los Angeles into a home in Three Points, AZ. Wow, that in and of itself would be a change. This girl had not known her current caretaker but the girl's mother knew the caretaker 15 years previously and thought it would be a good place. The girl, Cynthia, had lost both her parents to AIDS, it was not determined if she had AIDS, and her family was not a resource. Would Casa Gloriosa be a placement for her?

What a question. And there was little time to make a decision. I called Ken who said, "What's the worse that will happen? If we can't provide for her we'll call CPS but isn't this the direction we think the Casa is moving?" So we told the state employee that she could be placed at Glory House. Two days later I was called asking for an immediate pick up of this girl. CJ and I drove to a Circle K on the west side and met and took Cynthia and her belongings to Glory House.

I recall the first thought when I saw Cynthia, "Wow, she isn't very big. If she really is a handful I can sit on her!" I thought that with some relief. We had rumors of really tough behaviors and there was some trepidation on my part. Once settled in the truck on our way to Glory House CJ and I talked about Casa Gloriosa. He told his story and I talked about the rules and expectations of the house. Cynthia asked a couple of questions and indicated that she could and would abide by the rules. She even thanked me for picking her up. That caused me to wonder about her.

So, I asked, "Hey Cynthia, you now know who we are and what we expect. What is it that you want from me?"

Cynthia who has attitude said with a clear and strong voice, "Well, since you ask. I want to really know about the disease that killed my parents and that my sister has and I want to know if I have it."

"Okay, I can teach you about HIV and we will have a test completed on you as soon as possible. Is there anything else?"

"Yes. I have prayed for one year that God would send His angels and get me out of that hellhole, and you are a funny looking angel, but you came. I want you to know me the rest of your life."

"Well," I responded as soon as I swallowed the emotion in my throat, "I can't promise that but Cynthia I will find a good place for you to live." And so Cynthia Isabel came to Glory House.

At the time of Cynthia's admission there were six children and three adults in residence. She quickly fit into the daily routines, excelled at all expectations and expressed boredom in the school where she was placed. It was soon our thought that she would be placed in what seemed an ideal home of our friends. They were educated and had financial security and wanted Cynthia. So, weekend visitation was initiated and in that came resistance and eventually disclosures from Cynthia about her strong desire to not be moved out of the Casa. We used a therapist to evaluate her and learned that her IQ was 149 so she was moved into a more challenging school that really suited her. The therapist basically told us that the home would not work for Cynthia and that she had determined to be part of our life and either we needed to embrace her or move her far from us. Cynthia came to live in our home in March 1999.

Ken's words

I call her "Izzie" and she likes that, but then she likes me pretty much. I think she needed a dad and she likes our openness about my health and she enjoys my sense of humor. And, I didn't try to get her to like me. I've told Johna, these kids are coming into our world and we have to maintain it. If they aren't upset at us about once a week we probably aren't doing a good job at parenting. Cynthia Isabel has so much potential but I fear for the hardness of her heart. She loves me with all the capability of love she has, but without a stronger touch from Jesus her capability will not be expanded. So, the role of Casa Gloriosa in her life and the responsibility of Johna and me must simply be "to be Jesus to Cynthia for this season of time."

It has always been one of the most asked questions or curiosities, "How did you get it?" I did tell Johna when we first started this work, "We will not be offended." She says that is one of the principles that have allowed her to "having stood, stand." This question is one that pushes on me and I have to remind myself, "no offense." Johna and I determined that when questions or situations occur that could be offensive we would use them to teach. I think the response when a person shares his or her HIV status as a function of birth or blood transfusion is kinder than when the status comes from drug use or sexual behavior. I understand that and have said many times that most of us adults who are HIV infected have come to that status because of our misbehavior. I believe that. We make choices and there are consequences. That doesn't mean there should be harshness or refusal to serve the HIV positive drug user. I think of Casa Gloriosa as places where HIV infected or affected people are served regardless of the how or why. It is kind of like the person who is burned because he went to sleep with a cigarette in his mouth and is treated the same as the person burned because of an electrical dysfunction. The treatment is the same.

In writing this book I reviewed my notes and journals and found some writings when we were three years into knowing of my HIV positive status. I wrote, "Strangely it doesn't get easier. I remember the day that I found out I was positive as if it were yesterday." I told Johna that I felt lonelier than I ever had in my life, and I still feel that way sometimes. I am not a sullen or withdrawn individual and yet there have been times when I've had to make myself stay engaged. I see Johna fight against bouts of depression and withdrawal. And then there is the reconciliation that Jesus is the Great Healer and I am His child who is HIV positive and then HIV symptomatic and then with full-blown AIDS. What is the exercise of faith in this life situation? I know that I'm not being chastised and my walk with Christ does not hinge on whether He heals me.

Initially we read everything available to educate ourselves about HIV/AIDS; however there was a time that the information was troubling to me. I recall one visit, about three years into the disease, to the doctor's office. We discussed my symptoms and I noticed the doctor was not writing anything down. I was curious. She gave me some information and as I scanned it everything I had shared was included as a symptom of the disease in its progression. So, my doctor had only to check off a list of symptoms to know right where I was in the development of HIV toward full-blown AIDS. It is a little disturbing to read about your demise or the path that the "bullet" will take before it is fired. I went through a time when reading about the disease only added to my anxiety and paranoia so I stopped reading. It is different now. Now much of the reading confirms my position of not taking the medications.

I've thought and talked with Johna a lot about spiritual AIDS. There was a time I wanted to "give a lesson" about this starting with A = apathy. I think I had some anger with us as Christians that came out in my study and talk. Thank goodness that most of the words were only with Johna. We as Christians seem to be dying in terms of our love of Jesus. I never stayed true to Him until 1988 and I was a mere child when save and filled with the Holy Spirit. Many are the times I betrayed the Lord and many times He forgave me. Why wasn't I then satisfied to serve Him? The rebellion and selfish desires was my lord. At one point I didn't even know myself because of the distortions I allowed. In those days we, that is I, myself and me, never talked and I became dead in the core of my heart. So many of my friends with AIDS speak of feeling dead in their core, and then I spend time with my Christian friends and hear the same condition. In the early years of living with this disease I allowed myself to be beaten up about my culpability. For me sin, wrong decisions, and willful self-centeredness, played the major part in acquisition of HIV. However, God has worked a marvelous release and understanding of how He loves me. When He looks at us He sees Jesus. Because I am in Christ God does take what we have to offer, turns it inside out and uses it to His kingdom benefit.

Johna shares

We are faced with a decision. Ken's T-Cell count is down and his viral load is up so we must talk about his use of the medication. I know this is going to be a big decision for him and I know that his decision will be okay. We have seen the side effects of the medications, we have seen a lot of death, and we know that Ken's is not as healthy as he was a couple of years ago. We also know that in 1992 he was told to expect about four years of life and we should "do all we want to do in the next two years because the last two will be years of dying." Hmmm. That didn't work out like we were told. And, then in 1996 he was encouraged to start the medication and there was an implication that he might not live much longer if he didn't. He still lives and another year has passed. He is tired a lot, there is more often the smell of HIV and the symptoms seem harder to overcome.

Ken shares

I know my counts are not great and today we'll have to talk about the medications. Here is my position. There was the bout of projectile vomiting and severe diarrhea that lasted about one year. The naturopath figured out I had developed a dairy allergy and that pretty much cleared up. My neck and back has been painful now for about three years and I take some pain medication and even a muscle relaxer and that helps but I'd like to live without those pains. There is no bargaining with God. It is not, "Hey God if you will do this I will do that." However, I believe that faith comes by hearing and hearing by the Word of God and there is one goal in my life and that is to be a man of faith. I don't care as much about living or dying as I care that my life is one of courage to stand in faith.

The medical community talks about the medication as "the answer" and that is not the truth. It can help, but people on the medication will too die. I believe God numbers my days and not even my wrong decisions will shorten or lengthen them save suicide that is never part of my thinking. The routines and the noise of many people with AIDS are centered on the medication. It dictates life. My life is and will be dictated only by His truth. What can I do to help insure that I remain true to Him is of bigger concern to me than whether I have the "right" medication routine. And then I consider my heritage. My grandparents, my parents, the people of influence in my life are people who know and trust God and read His Word. If anyone should be able to stand in faith, believing and having peace that God is able and that He will do what is best, it ought to be me. Why not me? I am willing to be willing to be courageous and faithful to stand in faith that my days are solely and completely in You, O God. And that is how I came to decide that reading His Word daily, lots of it, in fact since 1998 about 21 chapters a day, would better serve me in this disease than the medications offered by the medical community. This is not the plan for anyone else and we are quiet about it not wanting to influence others to deal with AIDS in this manner. This is my journey with God and the other person most affected is Johna. She supports me in this decision. I decided on 21 chapters of reading per day because that was, at that time, the average number of pills our friends with AIDS were taking each day. The medication, this wonderful Word, has changed me. I still don't love enough, there are times when my faith isn't as solid as I want and there are days when all I can do is live but I am changed day by day to be more like Him.

Johna's words

Today the doctor plainly and clearly laid out the need for Ken to start taking the HIV medications. Maybe I was tired or maybe the reality of the progression of HIV in Ken's system hit me differently but I cried and cried. The doctor was flustered and I wanted to stop crying but finally just left the room. When I returned red faced and without make-up Ken was telling her that he did not plan to take the medication. She questioned him thoroughly and challenged that he wasn't thinking about me. At that juncture I had to inject that my tears and emotions were not to be taken as an indication that I was upset or disagreeing with Ken's decision. We left the meeting quietly. Ken talked with me as he drove so I could apply some make-up and get to work. The facts are startling and yet there is a sense of knowing that Ken's position is not one to prove anything but merely a statement, I think, of his trust in God. I wonder if there will be a time when I cannot eat or sleep but only pray for his healing. I have considered that if God heals Ken our life will certainly change again. But then, what's the worse that can happen in that kind of change!

Ken shares

At Camp Glory 1999 Johna and I did the daily HIV education and support group for the kids. It was fun and I think some of the teaching helped even me realize the relentless nature of HIV. For example, I made a "man" out of old clothing that I filled with dirt and straw. On this day of teaching I talked with them about "the other man". There are days, actually now about all the time, that the "other man" visits. It is as if another body is laid on me and everything, eating cereal, combing my hair or walking, takes too much energy. So the kids took turns having this "other man" strapped on their bodies and then walking around the group room just three times. The large teenage boy said, "That's nothing. I can run."

"Cool," I replied. "Why don't you run three times around the room?" I knew this young man had only months before learned of his dad's HIV status and I could hear some anger. At the end of lap two he was panting but he finished the third lap and as I helped remove the "other man" we had eye contact. The tears formed and then ran down his face as I embraced him. It was a great session as he talked about lacking understanding of how much it took for his dad to just do the daily stuff of life. When everyone left he walked the room again wearing the old man. He told me, "When I'm mad at my dad I will think of this the "other man". Thanks Ken."

Another day at Camp Glory 1999 I had the kids strap a bungee cord around their ankles and then pull it up a few times and/or pull the bungee cord across their chest several times. They quickly wore out and the point of fatigue was made to this group of kids of whom many will become a caretaker of sorts for their dying parent. We also talked about the joint pain and how it sometimes feels like pliers is being applied to the joint.

These days' people want to know about those who die of AIDS. I think it is because many people think I'm dying. Where's faith? The thing about AIDS death that still amazes me is how varied the dying moments are with one just falling dead of a heart attack and another wasting away until there is nobody left. Some die fairly quickly because of an organ failure or because of continued drug use. What? Why would someone with AIDS continue to use drugs? It is crazy isn't it? Yet many of our friends use drugs until very near the end of life. The typical look of a very ill person with AIDS is a hollow face, thin body, short or no hair and disjointed statements. As the end draws near many old friends stop visiting. One thing that bothers me for our dying friends is the lack of visits by relatives and especially by parents. I suppose this is because they can't come to grips with what is happening to their family member or friend. Yet, there are few honest talks about what's happening. I think the silence is tough and one reason many of our friends enjoy Johna during this stage is because she goes right into the topic of how are you really, are you near death, have you seen the angels? People need to talk. I do think that the palpable fear and the deep bouts of depression is part of what changes the features of our dying friends. Several of our dying friends have taken up the habit of a daily phone call with Johna where they give a report and she returns a word of encouragement. Johna tells me that often, when the end is very near, the dying person starts giving the daily word of encouragement!

Johna shares

Dora called us. Carlos is in the hospital very ill. I went to visit him and was distressed by the look of Carlos and by his high temperature that caused him to shake so hard the bed moved. Three days passed and everyone told us Carlos was dying and Ken and I felt CJ ought to have an opportunity to tell him good-bye. Cynthia, Ken, CJ and I all went for this farewell to Carlos. I held him to absorb some of the shaking in an effort to make the contact as pleasant as possible. Ken held on to CJ and we each said some words, prayed and let with tears run down our faces. We love Carlos. I went back and sat with him late into the night. Days passed and Carlos is now in intensive care. He is no longer shaking and is so peaceful. I talked with the personnel in the ICU and they were kind in allowing CJ to come into the unit for another good-bye to his dad. This was just CJ and myself and Carlos and it was sweet and Carlos opened his eyes though I'm not sure he knew that CJ was in the room.

Carlos is back in a nursing home, still living, and it is better than the first one where he was placed. I visit him a couple times a month and sometimes every day for a few days in a row. It depends on the resource within me that I can give away. CJ asked to not visit him until early 2002 when he asked to go see, "my dad." On the way he told me that he thinks Carlos will die soon. We are pleased that Carlos, with reminders, knows us. His face lights up as we spend a little time with him. I've taken a picture of CJ to leave in his room. As we prepare to leave CJ says, "We need to pray," and he holds out a hand Carlos and the other to me. Without a prompting CJ prayers, "Our heavenly Father, please touch my dad. If he needs to die be with him, don't let him hurt. We love you. Help us. Amen." Carlos and I wipe our eyes, hug and CJ and I leave the room. I wonder about the fact that Carlos still lives even though he does not recognize any one, can't care for any of his bodily needs, and is so thin and changed that he doesn't look at all like Carlos Guerra. This is a bit scary to me and especially because I love Ken and see the illness growing in him.

Our budget at Casa Gloriosa has been based on doing the best we can to do what we believe God asks of us, and then watching Him bring the money. The annual income has only been about $75,000 and that means there is very little money to pay employees.

The money comes from here and there. A couple of years ago we received a check for $30,000 from a person. Neither Ken nor I knew this man and I wrote a receipt/ thanks note and then called him. His statement deeply touched us. He said, "I admire your work and am not courageous enough to be involved in this kind of work, but I am giving to Casa Gloriosa believing that God will increase my faith and courage." It was two years after this gift before we met the man. He was sweet and humble. We pray God brings boldness, faith and blessing into this life. Another large single gift came from a family whose son died of AIDS and they gave enough money to pay a Camp Glory. Generally, the gifts have come from individual although there have been, as of Feb. 2002, four churches that have given regular support to Casa Gloriosa. The United Way of Tucson and Southern Arizona has given some designated money to the Casa plus we have received a couple of grants from them. The Southern Arizona AIDS Foundation paid some scholarships for the children to attend Camp Glory and paid a few weeks for some women to stay at Glory House. Our Firm Foundation has been very supportive to the agency both financially and in terms of consultation. As the agency is expanding and providing more services to children the budget too will expand. When children are in residence there must be competent adult workers and the ratio must meet, at a minimum, the standard of the State of Arizona. Also, as we fill Glory House with children the need for housing for women and for teenagers or young adults who are HIV+ will become an issue. We have been a grass roots organization that is now in the pains of growing up into a more sophisticated agency. As these transitions occur Ken and I are committed that the same loving atmosphere, the place of sanctuary and the personal involvement that define the work continue. There is a simple way to insure the work continues in the same manner and that is to keep a strong prayer covering, a Board of Directors full of God's Spirit, and high expectations of all workers whether they are employees or volunteers.

Ken shares

A change is coming to Casa Gloriosa and we don't exactly know what it will look like or when or how it will develop. But, as much as we knew that Casa Gloriosa was to be established we know that it is time for some changes. In the last few months we have been in contact with a woman who was given guardianship of a HIV+ 5 year old boy by his mother prior to her death from AIDS. This mother requested that her friend, the guardian, find a loving home that believes in Jesus Christ to take care of her son. A year has passed and no such home has been identified. I'm hoping that Casa Gloriosa will provide blessing and help in this situation. Johna learned from the Child Welfare League of America that there are several annual requests to them for placement, into a Christian milieu, of HIV+ children whose have parents dead from AIDS. We are one of few, if not the only faith based agency, that can provide this type of assistance.

Johna's words

Let me talk a little bit about these HIV infected and affected children. They are resilient, willing to take risks, familiar with difficulties and changes, and they are not, for the most part, people with a victim mentality. They are survivors. I believe that unless we take hold of these kids and give them a chance they will make their own chance and it will cost all of us a lot. I really believe that unless there is a strong intervention that brings choices and hope these children will be the young adults in the streets with a gun in our face. For Ken and me these kids are as much last chance people as their parents are or have been. What happens to them immediately subsequent to their parent's death and/or during that time period when the parent is dying makes the difference in their tomorrows.

Chapter Six: Our Move to Glory House

Ken shares

From the beginning of our thought to be involved, in service, with people who are HIV infected or affected we, Johna and I, promised one another some things we would not compromise. We promised that the service, the housing and programs would be good enough for our clients or friends and therefore good enough for us. We promised that we would absolutely not allow ourselves to become offended at our HIV friends, at our Christian friends, at people who ask hurtful questions or at other service providers. And, we promised that we would always partner with God. The problem of financial support we would leave in His arena. And, then we lastly promised that we would give our best to this work.

So, we appreciate the furniture, the linens, the dishes, the food and the paint for walls and new clothes washers and dryers that have been given to the agency. If you visit Glory House you will find a clean, nicely furnished and happy place. When Johna and I would visit there our scrutiny included, "Would we be comfortable living here?" Even when the rules for the residence were developed we tried to think of what we could stand if we lived in a shelter for infected and affected people. That kept the rules simple. This is a safe place. Therefore, no drugs or alcohol and no sexual behavior except between legally married people and no words or actions of violence. Basically the expectations created safety and there could be little tolerance for violation of these rules. Only three times did Johna have to request a person move from the house due to breach of the rules. In all the people that lived there we had only one time when we had to call the police to assist in a married couple to move out.

In 1999 Johna was so tired and not just physically but emotionally and spiritually. We were living on the west side in a three bedroom home that we loved, but now there are two kids living with us so it seemed crowded and full. Something had to change and as we reviewed our life it made sense that Johna take a job that might be less hours and less stressful though the money would be significantly less. So she resigned from CPS and became a consultant for another shelter system in the city. There were benefits for us in this move; however, the greatest was a clear understanding that even more change had to happen. So, we agreed to sell the house, get rid of any extra personal stuff and use the money to move ourselves into a position of little debt. By selling the house we not only reduced personal debt but would move into Glory House and, in due time, Johna would resign from the consultant position working for Casa Gloriosa for no salary.

Johna shares

I believe that one of Ken's greatest sacrifices was selling our home. We could have paid it off in another four years and he was eager for me to have some security, plus he loved the privacy of living way out west and the large yard on which the house set. This decision reminded me of Ken's great passion to represent Jesus to the community of faith and to the community of people living with HIV. And, it reminded me of Ken's great love of me. He was concerned about my health and the lack of time together. God is funny. The lot next to us, we had hoped to purchase it, sold and a family put a house on it such that our privacy was greatly impaired. This happened during the weeks we talked about whether to sell our home. It made the decision easier!

Glory House is cleaned and CJ and Cynthia's stuff is all moved in and a friend sent some workers and a large truck to move the rest of our stuff. It all fit in the one load. The only possessions of size, that we took was our sofa, the dining room table and chairs and our king size waterbed! The move started after Thanksgiving 2000 and by December 1st we were settled at Glory House. Looking back we are grateful that no one else lived there until January of 2001 when an adult woman moved in with us.

Ken shares

In December 2000 Johna's Mother died. She has spoken about this previously but it hurt my heart that we did not have the money to attend the memorial nor the resource to leave the children behind for the days it would have taken to go to Missouri. Johna went to the Casa Gloriosa Christmas party, which is always a big deal with food, a program and gifts and food packed in large black trash bags for the parents to give their children for Christmas. In fact the celebration was only 3 or 4 days after her mother died. And then we were able to shut the door at Glory House and take a few days with ourselves. CJ and Cynthia were each kind and concerned about Johna as she had some tears, some times of privacy and some times of talking and talking about Helen. Johna has the best of her mother's traits.

Johna's words

Cynthia hugged me today telling me she was sorry I felt so bad about my Mother's death. We talked about how much I loved Mother and she shared some about her mother who also died in the month of December. Cynthia told me she did not have the sadness I was experiencing and we talked about other HIV infected/ affected kids who have lost a parent to death. We agreed that a lot of the grieving happened months and perhaps even years before the death. Sometimes the parent is simply not around because of drugs or sexual habits and for some parents there are physically there but unable to function as a parent. I again felt gratitude for my parents and set it in my mind that I'd try to establish a place where kids, infected or affected, could get a taste of what it means to have a good, a better than average, an involved parent person! The concern for Cynthia grows in my heart as she allows me to see the damage done to her heart.

In April of 2001 I resigned from the consulting position and with more attention and seriousness took up the work of being the Director of Casa Gloriosa. An intern and I provided an after school program from January through May and I could now give more attention to that program and the parents of those 15 enrolled children. And then it was time to plan for summer and for camp. The days passed quickly and I tried to give more attention to Ken. We do a lot of HIV education in schools, churches and for other social service agencies. In the beginning Ken and I would do the education, but as clients wanted to be part of this and particularly the children we became a popular speaking panel. There were lots of those events in the spring of 2001.

The summer of 2001 was different. Ken's daughter, Bree, contacted him in October of 2000 and we bought her a ticket to visit us over the Christmas break of 2000. She is pretty and full of opinion and actions that remind me some of Ken. I loved her straightaway. She shared lots of her life issues, pains and joys. We all enjoyed that week and she decided to come to Tucson for the summer working with children during the summer program. We hired another young woman, part time, and the two of them worked hard to keep in contact, provide fun and help the kids get ready for camp. In July before camp Ken's health was obviously not good. In my opinion this was the biggest factor in Bree leaving before Camp Glory. Bree's visit was a good gift from God.

Ken's words

This summer my daughter, Bree, will spend time with us. She will work with the Casa Kids. I am nervous. Living here with us will not be like the week she visited and how am I to behave? Like a father or like a friend. Really there is no right on my part of "parent" her and yet I am, in fact, her father and it is my belief that she has missed some of what a father needs to give a daughter. Way back when I was in jail and Johna was in prison I spoke to a man about Jesus and that young man gave his heart and life to Jesus. Two years later at a youth camp he was a guest speaker and talked about me. My daughters were there. I think of how far God will go to keep His word and His promise to me is that my daughters will have an absolute and pure opportunity to know Him. I pray that the Spirit of God that once lived in their young hearts will be ignited and that they are restless until in Him they find sweet peace.

Johna's words

Bree's entrance into our life caused lots of rejoicing for Ken and me. Remember the list of 10 items we burned on our honeymoon? Well one of the items was for reconciliation between Ken and his daughters. Another daughter, Lana, had visited us a few years before, Ken was invited and attended her high school graduation and we felt that the relationship with Lana was okay, and now here was Bree. In the years of our marriage Ken and I worked to clean up old debts and wrongs and had done all we could to rectify any wrong toward his daughters and ex-wife. One of the experiences with Bree that I enjoyed was praying with her for her mother. And I know that Ken's words of respect about Bree's mother surprised and encouraged her. It has been an interesting process of Ken moving from a position of anger toward this woman to one of prayer that she would be reminded of God and His love for her. God is great at restoration.

Ken shares

Bree is pretty, quick witted and capable, and I believe God has great things for her if she will be willing to be willing! The pain, the victim mentality and the need within her can, in a second, be gone as she fully gives herself to Jesus. There are things that I'd have liked to have done better but the truth, as I understand it, about relationships, putting God first and living life with eternal meaning, Bree heard. Hopefully she and I will have yet another time of being together. The only item left on our list of 10 that we placed before God on our honeymoon is the publication of the writings and we have always believed the writings would be part of the financial support for Casa Gloriosa.

Johna shares

Harold, Ken's dad, came a few days before camp. Dear Lois knew that it was the year he must attend and we were so glad to have him be part of this tremendously emotional and uplifting experience. In those days Harold was with us at the house he and I realized that Ken was not able to go to Camp Glory and Harold agreed to stay in Tucson with him. The 60 campers plus workers including me left Glory House by 9:30 a.m. that Monday excited to get the hour and half south of Tucson to the camp location. It was a good day. We had the most competent counselors we had ever had for camp and many of the kids have attended every camp.

All day I carried a pain for Ken and so I called him late that afternoon. He told me that his temperature was 102 degrees. For Ken to take his temperature startled me and the reading concerned me. I called him early on Tuesday morning and knew he was very ill. So, I called our dear physician friend Mauricio. He went to check on Ken and immediately encouraged Ken to be admitted to the hospital. Mauricio took Ken and the process of admission was smoothed out by the doctor's order. Late on Tuesday I called to learn that Ken was admitted.

The day finished. At 9 p.m. I left Camp Glory knowing the workers were very capable and my husband needed me at home.

I admit that the first hour of travel back to Tucson I cried and then "got a grip" and arrived at 11 p.m. at St. Mary's hospital. Ken looked so little and frail lying in the bed. Of course the room requirements included wearing a mask and gloves. The doctors had not determined Ken's problem and thought he might have TB. He was glad to see me and we refrained from emotion. Ken was getting lots of medications to fight infection so I really thought he'd be significantly better by morning. After he was drowsing I left for Glory House.

Ken wrote these next few paragraphs in 1994 and I read it first when going through his writings to put this book together. It will give you an idea of how the diagnosis of HIV impacts a person.

Journal note from Ken

But for the heart monitor and the lung machine consistently rasping, soaking the air with a soft hiss, the room was very still. There were seven people gathered beside the figure on the bed. All were silent. The man on the bed was quiet too, now. One small woman seated beside the bed began to pray softly but audibly. Her hand clutched the hand of the man on the bed. A few in the room looked up, at her, and then at one another. A tall man with silver hair and slightly sloped shoulders stood, walked across the room and placed two giant hands on the praying woman's shoulders. His lips moved though he could not be heard.

"Fluff." That's what she had thought the first time she saw him. "Pretty but fluff. Empty. A jock by the looks of him." Lord that seemed forever ago. Johna hated hospitals and especially of late. How long had she and Ken anticipated the total collapse of his health? Eight, ten, fourteen years? What would happen now? Who would she talk with? Johna thought back to the time when she and Ken first married living in the mountains of Colorado. O how they talked. Ken had been so certain things would work out, that they wouldn't have to be separated. "What great faith or is his crazy," she wondered, "Or just naive?" Turned out, he was a little of all that! Things had worked out okay. But this, this was very near death? And the room listened as she prayed, "O God, touch Ken, heal his body and know that again I stand willing to be willing for your plan."

Johna's words

Ken was hospitalized on Tuesday morning and still on Thursday there was no definitive word of diagnosis. A biopsy of the mass in his lungs did come back showing no cancer. I took a walk and cried. And then the TB test can back negative and we celebrated no more masks and now people could drop by and visit him. His humor is back we knew by his teasing, "Johna, something's wrong with me. What wrong with me?" We laughed. We have heard so many of our friends with AIDS ask, "What's wrong with me?" We looked at each other and our eyes said it all, "AIDS!"

Ken was admitted to this hospital without insurance and as I met with the social worker, completed the forms and paid the initial $200 all my concern had to be given up to our Senior Partner, God. The state insurance kicked in and left us with only a few hundred dollars of debt. Plus Ken will have insurance for the next months and most likely, on this plan, until I'm again making fair market wages. I like our Boss, He is the Lord God Almighty and He is always on time and pays every bill without delay.

All the tests were done except a repeat and Harold and I sat downstairs in the hospital waiting, refusing to talk much because we were individually too full of emotion. Harold has referred, for years, to me as "My Johna" and his love is very strong toward me; however, Kenny is his son and that love, well you can feel it when the two of them are either together or speaking of one another. What's next? I found myself pacing the lobby and asking about the delay only to be assured Ken was okay. And then there was the doctor, this doctor is "the main HIV dude in the County". I've always liked him and many of our HIV positive friends are his patients. He saw me and crossed the room asking about Ken. I could feel the emotion in my throat and was grateful that a swallow or two suppressed it. He told me that he'd take Ken as a patient. I wanted to hug him but instead told him, "You know Ken has chosen not to use the HIV medications and I don't think he'll change his mind." The doctor already knew that little fact but expressed a willingness to serve Ken. I felt some of the load of concern shift and knew that we had another partner in this journey. It was interesting to me that we also spoke, that day, about Casa Gloriosa and the need for additional services to children. The doctor may never know but his words about the agency encouraged me at this point in time when it would have been easy to throw in the towel, so to speak.

Ken's words

I have a new doctor and you know I really like him. He knows what he is talking about and he is very respectful. In fact, I feel my face get red with this story but after the hospital time ended and we were at his office and he talked with me in some detail I spontaneously said, "I like you." Well we all were taken aback but he is very nice, and hey I do like him. He explained that I have Valley Fever and the medication he placed me on is way strong and might be reduced but is most likely a permanent addition to my daily life. He told us that had I not admitted it is likely that I would have died and that my immune system is pretty much shot so I'm not helping fight the Valley Fever. He changed the medications and I felt better within a day or two.

Johna shares

The kids are coming back from Camp Glory and I must be at the house to greet them all. So, Harold stayed with Ken that Saturday morning and I awaited all our camp friends. The excitement remained among them but there's a level of tiredness and it is always good to be home! Many if not all the kids made cards for Ken and they all gave me a hug, asked about Ken and told me they had been and would be praying for us. I recalled that the angels of children go before God every day and was comforted. Some of our adult clients went to camp this year for rest and as helpers. I really appreciated their concern and particularly one sweet mother and father called numerous times over the next months leaving words of encouragement and support. Thanks Ed and Kelly.

Ken came home from the hospital on the following Tuesday and he was weak "as water". His balance was off and his appetite not strong so I keep track just to make sure he eats enough. His fever is under control and if it climbs I am to take him straight into the doctor or hospital. We are so happy to have him home that the joy in the house overcomes the panic that could grow because he is weak, thin and shaky. I appreciate the prayers of Cynthia and CJ who thank God that "Ken is better" and as the weeks pass they notice and thank God that "Ken is eating more" or that "Ken was able to go to church today." The list of our thankfulness is long.

And Jenna visits. She is Leigh Anne's daughter whom we love so much. She is sensitive to Ken and has always been. In church she would look always for and give Ken a hug though that might mean walking all the way to the front of the church. Now, she pats Ken's cheek and rubs his whiskered face and sometimes hugs him very tight. We always feel she gives us a piece of heaven with her smiles, her many words and great energy.

In October a woman came from North Carolina to live and work a month with us. I found this restful and very helpful. She had thought Casa Gloriosa would be an internship forum for her daughter; however it became a work she needed to do for God.

In this month I gave Ken much more attention and again I was feeling concerned about him. One night I awakened to this sound that caused me, literally, to sit straight up in bed. I leaned toward Ken, and yes, it was coming from him. Was it the sound of death? I prayed and stayed awake a long time and then Ken was sleeping, quietly. As strange as this may seem I didn't talk with him about the sound and put it out of my mind until again, in the night, I awakened to the sound. The next time this happened I asked Ken about the sound. He laughed, "Johna that is my prayer language." When I quizzed him about what he was praying, he responded, "For the church." I knew that was true.

We have had the privilege to be part of situations, in the body of Christ, that cause us to know that we, the Believers, need a new touch of God. In 1988, in the mountains of Colorado, Ken wrote a collection of poems called BLESSED BELIEVER and the one titled Blessed Believer goes as follows.

> Blessed believer thou hast been shown things of God previously unknown.
> Acknowledging how precious His gift to thee realizing that His grace was free.
> Many things, though not understood, knowing that all His gifts are good.
> Learning much and growing strong promises, to keep all your life long.
> Blessed Believer his child you are, your light is seen from near and far.
> Don't worry for the things you've done, cleansed by the blood of God's own son.

We need Believers that are bold and I don't mean loud, not people with more noise but those who boldly speak Jesus. He is the Hope of this generation. The people with HIV/AIDS are an opportunity to be Jesus. They provide a place where God's people could not only be Jesus but also see Jesus.

In 1993 as Ken struggled with the HIV diagnosis he wrote a lot about the Church and for us, in that time period, it was writings for us.

In reviewing his writings I place the following in this book because it speaks about the condition of the Church and we are desperate that the Believers, all of us, become stronger and more able to form that place of sanctuary because we know there are many more with HIV to come. The Church is the group best able to be safety for hurting people. I often think we, the Believers in Christ Jesus, ought to rejoice, be thankful and get to work on behalf of people living with HIV and AIDS because it is a great opportunity. We must not let this opportunity pass us by.

Writing by Ken

We, the Christians, must speak Christ or stay silent and find ourselves in a cesspool of sin. We, the Church, have grieved his Holy Spirit by toying with carnal displays and fleshly exhibits and in that we diminish the reverence and power of the Spirit's activity within our ranks. Our energy goes to seeking lofty assignments and ascribing names to ourselves that place us above others. And we remain divided by prejudice and our ideas of right and wrong. We scatter. We are divisive and contentious and in that rebellion grows. God's nature is united and to unite. In the place of rebellion there is less God and the longer we live with less or without God the less we are like Him. Satan has been so long without God that there is "no good in him." And you know it is not a matter of how we feel or what we think or discern because that will not and cannot alter the Bible. We are a people with a spirit of self, we demand our rights and we create strife and disharmony.

Why are we so rebellious? We have compromised holiness for comfort, sacrifice for convenience and fellowship for mere civility. We lack obedience to God holding that we are worthy to decide what parts of the scripture matter and which portions we will apply into our daily living. We are rebellious because we lack the warmth that love produces. Not that hype or sugary pretentious dialogue we can all quote verbatim, you know the "I'm okay, you're" okay chit chat we all talk, but the informed conversations that are based in familiarity and mutuality. Genuine prayer does not take place unless we know one another. For there to be love there must be sharing. We as a group of Believers are not "sharers" but rather we cling to what is ours and often ignore the needs of those about us. We don't share emotions or behaviors because we don't trust one another. And we don't trust one another often because we don't trust ourselves.

And, we are rebellious because we refuse to be honest. We are not honest with ourselves so we cannot be honest with one another and there is no accountability. It is in that place that rebellion flourishes. We are not honest with ourselves because we are not honest with God. Honesty and truth will set us free; however, honesty and truth will only come as we immerse ourselves in His Truth, the Scriptures, and the Holy Word of God. Where honesty is lacking compromise rules and when compromise becomes the standard we will see no great move of God. In Revelation 3:1 John wrote, "Rouse yourselves and keep awake and strengthen and invigorate what remains and is on the point of dying; for I have not found a thing that you have done, any work of yours, meeting the requirement of My God, or perfect in His sight." [Amplified New Testament]

And then I share with you another poem from BLESSED BELIEVER that talks about what we, as believers, ought to be, begetting seed. And I pray and believe that the Casa Kids will become begetting seed. This poem is titled Begetting Seed.

Begetting seed, most sacred sown, the seed of Christ His very own.

Rooted deeply, planted firm unharmed by peril, storm or worm.

Rise up, Rise up Kingdom Seed
Begetting Seed, meet the need.
Scattered by a Holy Wind begetting seed will rise again.
Look around for the hungry need; we are Jesus' begetting seed.
Rise up, Rise up Kingdom Seed
Begetting Seed, meet the need.

Johna shares

By the first of November Ken was not a lot better and I felt weak and weary. So, with Ken's agreement, I called about 27 people of faith asking for a meeting at Glory House. We told them that Ken's T-Cell Count was 43 and his viral load more than 750,000 per little bit of blood. A healthy T-Cell Count is 1200 and a person without HIV has no viral load since that tells you the amount of HIV per little bit of blood. Obviously Ken's counts were not good; he slept many hours a day and had not gained a lot of weight back from the 20 pounds he lost before and during the hospital stay. It was a good time of fellowship and we shared some of our burden with this special group of people. I asked for 21 days of prayer inviting people to stop at Glory House and we made room for such gathering. I left a book for people to write their prayers, comments or thoughts to Ken and me. Many people came during those days and one woman wrote beautiful prayers based on scripture to us every day via e-mail. Ken got better. He gained about 10 pounds, his hair grew back, he was able to be awake and up more during the day, and he is on a different Valley Fever medication.

People ask, "Is Ken healed?" This question takes me back to a time early in this disease when he was vomiting every day and often it was a projectile vomit that really made a mess. We were invited to speak on PARENT TALK and were flattered and nervous to have such an invitation. Ken had to go with me. He agreed. We prayed, got dressed and started the drive to the radio station. At least three times in that drive we had to pull over and Ken vomited. When we arrived he was gray, sweaty and shaky. "Ken, I'll explain. Can you wait in the lobby or restroom?"

"Give me a minute first," Ken replied.

As I waited a few minutes in the lobby I thought of God's power and prayed He would touch Ken. "Hey, I'm really okay." Ken returned from the restroom where he'd washed his face and touched up his hair. He looked okay. We completed the radio show, left the studio going home and, sure enough, we had to pull over a couple times on the way home. That is healing. Ken had the strength and ability to keep his commitment that was in the best interest of God's work. I hold on to that example and believe that Ken can do anything that he needs to do for God. God says His strength is made perfect in our weakness and over and over I've seen that promise made fact in Ken's life.

More than once I've been asked, "Are you fasting and praying for Ken's healing?" Maybe there will be a time when I can go away from the day to day of life and the work of Casa Gloriosa to focus on Ken's healing. However, I really believe Ken's days are numbered and nothing, not our wrong decisions, not taking or refusing the medication and not the amount of fasting and prayer I give will change that fact. I trust in God for Ken's life. "But what about asking and seeking and knocking?" some ask? I do ask and seek and knock for a touch from God in Ken's health. I love my husband and God knows that there is in me a willingness, at least a willingness to be made willing, to experience the changes that will occur if Ken dies or if he is healed of AIDS.

Ken shares

We miss our two friends that died in December of 2001 of AIDS. Johnny was a good guy, kind, and he loved Jesus. The last couple years of his life he often spoke of his church and his Pastor John whom he really loved. He was sitting in his chair and died. He didn't have to be back in the hospital or suffer days and weeks in pain. He died. And then a mother died leaving two teenage girls. This woman was a friend for five years and we miss her. Many days in the last month she'd call, in the morning, and leave a word of encouragement for us. If Johna answered the phone she always asked, "Johna how about a prayer for the day?" In the summer she and I spent some time together and she told me later, "I will wait for you and Johna in heaven by the flowers that have red stems." I had told her about my dreams of heaven.

I asked Johna, "Who were those men? They were dressed really sharp in black suits and they were beautiful?" I was confused that she didn't seem to know whom I was talking about. A day or two later I asked her again about them. They were at our house, but she didn't see them, at least she can't remember. Then at the funeral of our dear friend who left the teenage daughters I realized the two beautiful men were angels that came to assist our friend home to heaven. As I told Johna, during the memorial service, about the angels the tears flooded my eyes and ran down my cheeks. God is so good to me. He lets me know some things. It has been a couple of years past that I had such beautiful dreams and I know I experienced a bit of heaven. In fact it was fun to talk with Helen, Johna's mother, about these dreams. She was closer to heaven than we realized back then; however, she had sensed heaven near her and our sharing was comforting to each of us. Maybe my dreams are not of the literal place but they bring a sense of peacefulness and joy deep in my spirit. There is no fear in me of dying. The question is whether it is better for Him if I remain or if I go? He knows.

In one dream I saw the most beautiful water. It was of different colors and some was running up and other bodies of water ran down, and fish in it were splendid in shape, size and color. The plants in this land were exquisite. And you know there was no bloom dying. The roses were awesome and full, some were in bud but none were dying and there are no dead flowers, leaves or sticks anywhere. The colors of the plants were more than I could comprehend. It was a place where the smell and the sound made me want to touch and taste and rest forever and ever.

Chapter Seven: So What Have We Learned?

Ken shares

They told me I don't have much time and that's pretty much a given outside the power of God. But you haven't read this book to just hear another horror story about a rebellious youth. It hasn't been my plan to tell such a story. What I will say, "Whatsoever a man sows that shall he also reap." If you take risks in life, make poor decisions, waste yourself recklessly; you can be sure that there will be a payday. But thankfully, when you come to the end of yourself you find Jesus. Several years ago Johna and I began to ache for the wounded around us. We sought God for direction and for years never knew what specific group would be our task, but we knew there was a task, you know? We knew and God surprised us along the way in little and big ways and He showed us clearly that the reason we could not sleep or eat or talk of anything else was because of His stirring. We prayed, we hoped.

God is a God of mystery and wonder and it is a wonder He was so very patient with me. Then one day, challenged by a friend I tested for HIV. It came back, three times, positive. And we knew. Our goal has been to provide an atmosphere of love and comfort to people with this horrible disease. Paul might call that reasonable service.

The Lord said that His yoke is easy and His burden light. Then what is it that sometimes threatens to press us into the ground and break our hearts? Remember the Lord's command? He said, "Take up your cross and follow me." What is a cross? It is shame, public humiliation, guilt, stress, and consequences. Who fashions our cross? We do. Jesus yoke is easy but the cross, we bear the cross we built for ourselves and the weight of it will be crushing unless we allow it to be fitted into the yoke He prepared for us. Johna talks about this process in terms of stones and she needs to write that book.

Casa Gloriosa, like the yoke placed on Johna and me, is still being fashioned; still being shaped and we ask that you join with us in extending to those with HIV/AIDS the hand of fellowship, the hand of healing and the hand of love. It is so good to be part of this work. Over and over I have been amazed. We have met people we could never have know, been invited to memorial services, birthdays and several churches where they call us friend. I know that God is well pleased with our efforts. I pray that the next days of Casa are as purely motivated as the beginning. As long as we are faithful to the vision we hold, God will honor the work with support financially, with health enough for the tasks and encouragement directly from His tremendous heart of love. We don't really know how long Casa will remain active, supported, filled with people and of course children, but that is up to our Senior Partner, God Almighty. We do know that change is coming.

Johna and I spent three weeks in a cabin, thanks to a friend, putting this book together. We talked more honestly about my health. What's up with my loss of balance and the fact that sometimes it is difficult to read because of my eyesight. In these days of being at the cabin my health has declined. Johna holds me. AIDS destroys self-image. Whatever I thought I was changed with HIV diagnosis, and as there are more symptoms and AIDS takes a stronger hold I feel like life is done and that I don't even know me. There is peace deep in me. I touch Johna's face often and tell her that change is coming. Then I consider the words of Proverbs 24:10: "If you faint in the day of adversity your strength is small." I will not faint. I have Jesus.

We, the Believers, do not have to settle for what man can devise as help. Recall Peter, the Apostle, in a small boat being tossed and thrown by the winds and waves. In the midst of fear and anxiety, cold and wet and scared Jesus came. The men in the boat saw Him and failed to recognize Him until Jesus called out, "Be of good cheer. It is I; do not be afraid."

Peter calls out, "If it is you command me to come to you on the water."

Jesus simply said, "Come".

Despite adversity, set backs or confusion I will focus on Jesus rather on the mighty waves or the threatening winds. I will remember what Peter forgot for only an instant: between my Lord and me there is nothing but solid ground. The reality of that truth is all I can see as my eyes stay fast on Him.

Johna shares

Of this I know Ken is a strong man in the spirit. His body is weakened and there are moments that I freeze, some moments, and more than friends understand, when tears flood my eyes, and once in a while I let myself consider his death or his healing. There is no middle ground in this situation. Ken will either be healed or he will die and according to his counts that will not be long from now. The doctor was clear at our last meeting. The viral load is a number of HIV replication per milliliter of blood and there are, I think, 6000 milliliters of blood. So, Ken's viral load is higher than 800,000 times 6000 and that's a lot of HIV. When I paused to recognize this number the situation is beyond what I can understand, and in that place I have a different kind of peace with God. I know Ken did not take the position of no HIV medication to prove a point. He trusts in God and believes that the journey, trusting in God, will be best for him, for me and for the work to which we've been called. I trust in Ken's faith and decision on this matter. I plan to spend more time with Ken, to insist on more great talks with him and to listen to his sleeping sounds, his thoughts and his needs, and to respond to him with respect and all my love. In these weeks putting this book together I know change is coming. Ken will either be healed or he will die. When there is a change I will rely on God who has promised that His strength is sufficient for all my needs.

Casa Gloriosa is an agency that is growing up! In the three weeks we have spent putting this book together we have also talked and prayed about this work that we've been given to oversee. What a joy and what a responsibility. We recalled that when Glory House opened it sat from November 1996 until April 1997 with no women admitted and we wondered and others wondered and yet we knew that the work was God's. It is time for change that some will say is not a need and others say the need is too great and too expensive. All we can do is trust His Spirit in us. The big picture, the ultimate goal, remains the same. There must be sanctuary for people who are HIV infected or affected. To us sanctuary means there are agents [strong Christian people] who stand arms linked creating a safe place, a place that stands against the forces [stress, drug use, bad decisions, lack of money for needs, broken relationships] that cause eternal death. Sanctuary is kind and welcoming and always ready for the person who needs it. In these, almost 14 years, I have learned deep in my mind and spirit that GOD IS. What a simple thought and yet everything in my life hinges on that truth. If God is then it is His way that I seek. If God is then it is His kingdom that I care about and His will that must be followed regardless of what seems like a cost. Because God is there is a way that is beyond any I can imagine or plan. In these years I have learned that to be courageous merely means that one must try and fail and try again. And it is not difficult to be courageous because the failures, in Christ, will become opportunities for His strength to be made clear and perfect. I have learned that people are discouraged and lonely and that is a condition best addressed spiritually. That children are not valued is a tough realization that I've learned in these years. Rarely do parents, our friends with AIDS or our Christian friends, make decisions based on what is in the best interest of the child. It is much easier to function in the mode of what's convenient for me, the parent.

I thought, years ago, that Ken was my love and my lovely husband, and I believed that in Ken "what you saw is what you got." I really liked and hoped that to be true, but in these years of living with him I have come to know that he is, in fact, my lovely husband whom I love and he is what you see. Ken is a man with an opinion and he is bold in the expression of it because all his opinions are based in his reading and understanding of God's word, the Bible.

In these years I have come to believe that everyone of us will be given stones. They are, my friend, precious stones that will either crush you or upon which you will fall and be humbled and broken so that you can learn obedience to the calling of God. This precious stone has felt like panic in my throat, a heavy weight on my back, rocks in the pit of my stomach and sharp edges in my heart, and I thank God that He has trusted me with such a stone. I am resolved to allow this stone to continue in me the good work it has begun.

Ken shares

When I recently had the bout of Valley Fever my body was ravaged and I lost weight and many believed, "this is it, Ken can't live much longer." I've never believed that was the case in this bout of Valley Fever and I was not and am not afraid of death. For those of us who serve "the least of these" in society there is much joy when one lost comes home. We do not enjoy the pain and shattered lives we've seen, but God is so faithful and we love partnering with Him who waits even at the door of death to welcome another home.

My health remained pretty much the same these years of living HIV+ and then with AIDS until the Valley Fever battle. I have been really healthy the past 14 years. I still refuse the AIDS medication and I doubt that my mind will change on that issue. When I think about this position the face of my good friend Mauricio comes before my eyes. We share from the core of our humanity and out of the Spirit of God that dwells in us. I love him. He never speaks to influence my thinking; he is a physician with God's healing power in his hands. I am pretty confident that Mauricio is glad to be the friend of a man who believes and therefore stands in faith. It is good to live by the convictions that resonant from your spirit. Sometimes God's presence is so near and there is nothing I'd exchange for any one of those moments. God is good and very real to me.

If you take only one or two things from this book let it be that God's provision will never fail you. I think that God gives each of His children an opportunity to bless someone else. It may not be hands on, or wallet on, it could be prayer but God puts a tiny seed in the life of His child and watches to see the reaction. Many of the opportunities, we often refer to them as situations, are kicked aside, crushed or never even recognized as from Him. I believe that most churches, a lot of pastors and yes even the musicians are plagued with "good enough" character that allows them to relax. I call these maintenance Christians, those who will hold on to what they have, but have too little to evangelize. Jesus is the model we have to follow. He may not have tapped you for AIDS ministry but Jesus has tapped all of us to service.

The joy of obedience you'll discover is more priceless than gold. I don't mean to say that Johna and I have everything figured out or that we've done everything correctly, far from it, but this we have learned: Jesus loves, Jesus loves, Jesus loves.

Chapter 8: So, What's Next?

Johna shares

We left the mountain to return to Tucson believing this book was finished and the next phase would be one of change and wonder and impact. Ken was ill all the way down the mountain. There was a message that a friend wanted to talk with us about a research treatment for AIDS. Ken was better late that day and I asked if he wanted to hear about this treatment. It surprised me that he agreed saying, "These friends are trustworthy. If they think we need to hear about it, okay." So a meeting was scheduled and Leigh Anne agreed to attend. It was my thinking that if the treatment sounded good I might need her input to influence Ken. Leigh Anne is one of few people with this kind of influence on Ken Reeves! We listened to the presentation and Ken was too ill to talk about it. As I put him to bed there was the reminder that, "Johna change is coming. You may need to call Dallas for help. But remember, God just might touch and heal me at the very last moment!" Ken laughed. His joy at life and his humor felt like warm soothing oil.

At 6 a.m. the next day I looked up from working on the computer to see Ken standing at the office door. He told me not to get up and with an empathetic tone spoke words that ring in my mind to this day. He said, "Johna listen to me." He held his hand palm up pointing a finger from the other hand to make the point, "God has numbered my days. Don't forget that Johna. God has numbered my days and He holds them in His hand. I'm going to do this treatment. It is not for me. It is for others and for you and for the Casa." He sat down and smiled. What could I say? As he drank some juice I encouraged him that the treatment was not necessary, that he could use the traditional medication or he could continue with no HIV medication. Tenderly Ken held my face in his hands and said, "Johna you are not listening. My days have been numbered and they are held in God's hand. This treatment is for others. It doesn't cause me spiritual angst. In fact I am not agreeing to this out of my mind but from my spirit. I'm going to do it. Call 'em up!"

Early in March Ken started a treatment with Dr. Sam. The day of the first injection Harold and Lois were in town. Ken had to be driven to several clinics for various tests and he and I went alone. We had great emotion and sweet calmness. He was very tired when we returned home. The base tests demonstrated the destruction of AIDS and Valley Fever in his body. He could not see good enough to read, his motor skill responses were all very poor, and he could not walk a straight line nor stand without weaving. This man who was known for strength, a devastating punch, endurance and quickness of wit was so small, weak and slow that Harold and I stood aside with tears threatening to drown our hearts. Two injections were given and the team told us that he would have a positive response within about 20 minutes. Harold and I still laugh as we recall the eye contact exchanged between us. We were on alert ready to end this charade and protect Ken. In less than 10 minutes Ken sat up straight and looked at me. I went immediately to his side and he laughed. The fullness of the laugh made me know he was better. Every test had improved so dramatically that he went outside and threw a basketball with CJ. The next morning Ken was up by 6 a.m. and wanted food. He ate with the family; the kids went to school and about 10 a.m. he wanted biscuits and gravy. I took him to a favorite restaurant. As Ken ate tears ran down his cheeks. He was so pleased to taste the pepper in the food. It had been more than two years since he had really tasted anything. As the meal neared an end Ken started moving his arms one-way and then another and stretching and frankly acting weird. Again the tears fell in sheets from his face and he said, "Johna there is no pain." You can only appreciate this comment if you have watched the person you love suffer every day for years with pain and the treatment that "might" work to end the pain we could not get because the insurance would not cover it. He had suffered much pain. Now, after one treatment the pain was gone and it remained gone. The deep appreciation and gratitude in our heart for Dr. Sam's work is without a venue of expression.

March and April were wild months! Another friend and his wife from our church came every day and gave Ken injections or merely checked up on him. Ken became dehydrated and had to have an IV and he fussed about it but the team made it fun using a rather fancy light pole from which to hang the IV bag. There were days in those months that Ken seemed very young and innocent and our sharing touched on the deep secrets and thoughts and delights that too many times people never share because of a lack of trust or time or hope. His eyesight was much improved but we developed the habit of me reading the Bible to him. What precious hours of reading and discussing. Many times in those weeks Ken prayed for me out loud while holding my face in his hands. And there were days Ken was very much the husband and parent. He spoke with authority and power and I believe understanding that came from God's Spirit.

Two themes of discussion developed in these weeks that have significant influence on me in this season of my life. First Ken talked a lot about "change is coming Johna." He was vague about the nature of the change but very firm that it was coming and he would often pat or hold my face and say, "It will be better. You are okay." And the other theme was about CJ and Cynthia. The discussion about these children was difficult for Ken and me because we disagreed and yet it was great because he was well enough to be part of making a decision that was really big. We came to an agreement that Cynthia had received all that we had to provide for her. We further agreed that there were issues that needed to be addressed in the context of her birth family. I made many contacts with her family of origin in California and a plan was developed that she would spend the month of June with her family there while CJ was in Nebraska with Harold and Lois. Ken and I further agreed that late in June I would go to California and develop with the family of origin a plan for Cynthia to remain in their care.

Harold started calling Ken on a daily basis in 1999 and sometimes in these weeks they would talk a couple times a day. Ken's love of his dad was an anchor in his life. Days when Ken didn't feel like moving he would because if he spent time in the word God would give him a thought for Dad. The faithfulness of Harold in his walk with God was a standard that Ken pressed toward. It is my recollection that Ken let Lois know how he loved and appreciated her in our life and especially the impact she has on Harold. In these weeks of good health Barb, Ken's mother, visited. I honor Barb that she was sensitive to Ken's need for affirmation from her. He needed to hear and she clearly told him that she was proud of his work in the community of people living with HIV/AIDS and in the community of faith. The times of reminiscing about days past were fun and good for Ken.

Ken said one day to me, "You know that Bill…" Ken was referring to his cousin and on the third time he spoke the same words about Bill I wrote them down. This started a fun exercise for me. Ken would say something like, "Let me tell you" or "Did you that that Dad" and I would write whatever he said. In the months from November 2001 until May 2002 Ken spoke about 27 men and 4 women. Interesting to me and I've given most of the people the words he said about them.

Ken's response to the treatment was fabulous. The Valley Fever was gone and could not be "grown" in samples of his blood again. The HIV counts improved and he was doing great. Ken talked with me privately about his thinking processes. Ken's mind was very good. He was quick, full of information and so creative in processing facts that he was a natural winner at debate. He had concern that physically he was better but that his thought processes were declining. In our years of marriage we requested few promises from one another. Ken requested that I stop the treatment if his mind became impaired to the point he made little sense or was unable to live in the now. I promised.

Ken's thinking and mental abilities did change. Actually his thinking had been changing for many months but our lifestyle kept it, for the most part, unknown. We, Ken and I, talked about it in terms of his mind having lost the screening filter! In other words, when a thought came into Ken's mind he merely said it. There was no processing of how it would impact another or whether the timing was best or if the words would better be heard with less of a crowd. Honestly, I liked this pithy and honest flow of thoughts from Ken. An example is a continuing word to me that will challenge me the rest of my life. Ken said, "Johna you know God's word is truth and life. It never returns void. I am reading and have for years read mega doses of His word so in heaven I imagine there will be a place of authority for me. All this word in me will continue to be used in eternity." What a great thought and I agreed. "Johna, you on the other hand," Ken says, "You are not reading enough of His word to get any position higher than something like bathroom cleaning. You've got to read more." His words came from his heart and his heart was full of God's word and Spirit.

On May 31st, 2002 some friends took CJ and Cynthia to Phoenix to the airport. Early that morning Ken awakened me and I helped him shower. He asked that I "put a little more of that cologne on me because the kids need to leave with the good smell of me." Breakfast was fun and full of excitement as they got ready to go. CJ had earlier in the week dreamed that he left and Ken died. It was precious to watch and hear Ken facilitate CJ's understanding that maybe the dream was God's way of preparing CJ for Carlos [CJ's birth dad with AIDS] or Ken's death but it was not God asking CJ to stay home. Ken was good with teaching the kids. One time Cynthia was sad because of rejection from her birth family. Ken had us all to the back room and he turned off the light. He flicked on a flashlight and talked about the beam of light from it. He probably had 10-12 flashlights and some beams were small, some a bit yellow, and every beam was different. He piled them all in a heap leaving the light beam turned on. He told her, "Izzie sometimes there comes a light so bright and beautiful and different that it is simply too much for the crowd where it shines." He turned on a huge bright beam from some work light and told you, "You are a bright light that could not, at the time your family put you out, understand. You are bright and beautiful and there is a plan for you that is wonderful." Izzie loved Ken a lot.

As they kids start to walk out the door Ken says with a finger pointing toward them, "Hey, I'll see you in a month or in heaven." They froze. CJ ran and threw himself on Ken who hugged and teased him and Cynthia stood looking at Ken. He said, "You know if anything happens to me I will be in heaven and I expect to see you there. It is up to you." CJ always loving and responding to Ken, "Yep Poppa, I'll be there. But we'll see you in a month."

The kids are gone, the house is really clean and we have stocked up on fun food and anticipate privacy! Ken asks if we can pray through the house, Glory House. It was sweet and God's presence seemed to fill the spaces and we commented on feeling rested and appreciative of this time alone. Ken's mom stopped in and Harold called, the doctor checked Ken who had a UTI but was "doing great", and we kept the blinds drawn enjoying privacy. At one point on Friday I noticed Ken craning his head as if he saw someone down the hall. After a couple times of noticing this I asked Ken if he saw something or what? "Oh Johna you don't see them?" Ken laughed and laughed. No I didn't see anything but was alerted that something was up with Mr. Man Ken!

"Johna," Ken said, "the angels are here."

"Ken Reeves," I immediately responded, "What are angels doing here?"

He laughed, "I don't know. They are either here to minister to me or to take me home." I prayed immediately that God was touching Ken's body by the presence of angels and that Ken would have perfect health. We were close in spirit and proximity that day. Ken was some uncomfortable because of the urinary tract infection and always feeling like he needed to void but it was a good day. Friday night Ken was asleep by 9 or 10 p.m. and I stayed in the bedroom reading until I could sleep.

Early Saturday morning Ken awakened. He was wide-awake and it was 1 a.m. so up we got and he ate and we watched all the old Casa movies and news reports. It was fun and we felt that life could not be better. For several of those early hours we read the Bible, reviewed our story and God's grace. Ken loved to tell me how amazing he found it that God brought us together and to remind me how much God loved a woman named Johna. We looked through this manuscript reminding ourselves of life and I read a few letters from prison and we were again stunned at the level of intimacy and sensuality we shared in every piece of our life. I read some of the poems Ken wrote for me over the years. He talked about the gift of writing and the creativity of his person. He told me that one of his best life experiences was writing THE VIAL SO PRECIOUS because he felt, smelled, heard and lived the story. A big compliment Ken gave me that early morning was his statement that "there is no story I'd rather be a participant in Johna than the story of us in God." We talked about the love of one another and the sadness we feel because most never experience such love. We prayed words of thanksgiving and spent time talking with God about the people who were part of Ken's medical team. The team was Dr. Sam, Michael B., John & Bobbi V., and Mike P. with Mauricio as our private word to confirm that the decisions we made were within the realm of reasonability! We are people that do not believe in coincidences so these men and their wives were brought into Ken's life for reasons bigger than Ken "getting better."

Sometime on Saturday Ken took a ring I'd given him off and asked if I hold it for him. He denied it bothered him but said, "I don't need it anymore." This caused me to consider that he had taken his earring out giving the same statement a few weeks earlier and that he stopped drinking coffee some weeks prior to that giving the same statement. So, I asked Ken about all these statements and if the angels were still at the house and I asked him if he was going to die. The look he gave me was priceless and he laughed. "Johna change is coming and it is good."

We were up about 1 a.m. on June 1st and finally about 9 p.m. Ken lay down to hopefully sleep. A friend, Andy Stang, stopped by and his presence calmed me. When he left his concern caused him and his wife and some others to pray for eight hours of rest for Ken and me. They stayed in prayer for a length of time until it seemed they knew that rest was in the house of the Reeves. Once Ken was resting I showered and came to bed about 11 p.m. Ken opened his eyes and said, "Hug me."

"Oh Ken, here lay on my arm," I insisted and we lay face to face with his head resting on my arm. We slept until about 1 a.m. when a noise awakened me. Ken was laughing. I mean the man was really laughing from deep in his belly. I rose above him looking at his face that was so happy. Hearing the laughter I prayed thanking God for giving Ken rest and peace and that, by the look on Ken's face, he was feeling ever so much better. Thank you God!

Ken would mumble and then laugh. I asked what he laughed about and he'd pat my head and face and mumble and laugh some more. From 1 until 5 a.m. he laughed and mumbled with one sentence clearly being, "I've got to go over there." As for me, I rested speaking words of gladness that God's touch to Ken was one of healing. Deep in my spirit I felt preparation. Ken was better, life would change and as Ken kept saying, "It will be good."

At 5 a.m. I told Ken my arm hurt and I needed to move. As I helped him get repositioned I thought he felt heavy but he quickly went to sleep and I too slept until about 6:45 a.m. when Katie Belle, our loyal bull terrier, awakened me. I heard Ken sleeping but said, "Ken I've got to let the dogs out, don't get up." He did not respond and I quickly got up and walked around the huge waterbed to his side.

Ken was beautiful. His face was rested. He opened his eyes as I neared him and they were pools of blue full of light, and his smile drew me near him. His arms embraced me and we kissed and then I kissed his face several times and he patted mine. "Oh Ken you are resting so good. Don't get up," I told him as I put my face against his.

"Johna it is so beautiful I'm going to sleep some more," Ken smiled at me.

"Thank you God for touching Ken. Rest Ken. Don't get up. I'll be right back," and I patted him. The two dogs quickly were put outside; I brushed my teeth with a quickness and thought how good a cup of coffee would smell but wanted first to check Ken making sure he rested.

I entered the bedroom, walked to end of the bed and turned right to check Ken. As I turned he opened his eyes and we had eye contact, he formed a smile that caused me to remain paused and then he closed his eyes and died. It was June 2nd, 2002 at 7 a.m.

Ken had talked so much to me about the Holy Spirit. "Ah Johna you must partner with the Spirit of God. Jesus is in heaven but the Spirit, He is your partner here. Johna, talk to the Spirit. And if I die pray making sure God doesn't want to raise me back to life." So, I went to Ken putting my hands on him and prayed, "Spirit of the living God I think Ken has died. You know. I ask for your life-giving touch to Ken. You are God and if Ken's continued living is your will cause him to live." I waited and looked at Ken. He looked so at peace and in the bedroom the pink mist of God's Spirit was present. In that place of sweetness I asked God to give me grace and power to represent Ken's life in ways that brought honor and glory to God. I thanked God for this man, this altogether lovely man who lived what he talked and had died in the glory of God. I thanked God for the impact of Ken's life on me and so many other people.

At about 7:10 I stated to Ken that I thought he had died but in case he had not I told Ken that I had to get the cell phone to call the doctor and then I'd be right back. After returning to the room I called the doctor who was stunned. He and his wife would be to the house quickly. Ken was modest and always looked good. I checked to clean him but there was nothing to clean. So I waited.

People that had position in Ken's life came. Harold and Lois were on their way to Tucson. Ken had instructed me to learn from Dr. Sam if an autopsy was needed so we waited. Mauricio came soon and he told me there was no smell. Eventually we learned an autopsy was not needed. At about 12:30 p.m. I turned on the music that Ken listened to over and over the last two months of his life. Brian gave us the CD and Ken called it the sound of heaven. The words start, "Now is the time for true worshippers to praise the Lord…"

The music was loud and they took Ken's body dressed in Calvin Klein jeans, a handmade shirt from Africa given him by Mauricio, white socks and a LA Dodger ball cap. I asked the doctor, then a friend and then I prayed. What else could we do?

Sanctuary, a safe place because God's people stand arms linked against forces that damage, has been extended me. People from every phase of Ken's life attended either the memorial in Tucson or the one in North Platte, NE. Our pastor John Aker and Rose, his wife, traveled to Nebraska so Pastor Aker could speak at the memorial. His words honored Ken. I don't think John Aker realizes the impact he had on Ken. Pastor Aker affirmed Ken's faith. He recognized that Ken was always, even 14 years after his commitment, in love with Jesus. Ken told me that when he thought of John Aker he felt himself straighten and be renewed to never give up.

Following the service in Nebraska, a Christian couple provided a home for CJ, Cynthia and me and we moved out of Glory House. This house and the location of it have helped us heal. Ken loved the desert and we live way out in it so talk about Ken is as natural as stepping outside or watching the quail from the window. Our decision that we had nothing more to give Cynthia proved true. My process in taking Cynthia to California was not the best but it was all I could do at the time. God is good and a Christian couple is helping to give Cynthia her next step. Cynthia needs both a mom and a dad and this family provides that for her. I bless them.

CJ attends a Christian School in our new neighborhood and a young Christian couple is teaching him to ride a horse and rope calves! He asked about Casa Gloriosa the other day and we ended up talking about a "normal lifestyle". His response was, "Mom I can hear Poppa saying, 'normal lifestyle for a Christian isn't good'". What can I say? We are not destined to live by the standards of this world. We are radical in our belief that GOD IS! CJ's birth dad, Carlos, died in December and again John Aker officiated at the memorial service where about 150 people came. Most of the people attending were folks from the church who had never met Carlos. CJ experienced healing as he sat among the people knowing, as he later told me, "Mom they came because they love me." Love is powerful and it heals. I bless the people of Christ Community Church who have taken time to learn about HIV and the impact of this disease on children. The college and career group from this church have assumed the responsibility for Camp Glory 2003. God is good.

The Board of Directors of Casa Gloriosa, since June 2nd, 2002 is made up of four people brought together for this time. I honor them. Brian Lynch stepped into the work of Casa Gloriosa because we needed help that required change. We trusted Brian and believed his skills would take the work to the next level and it has but that level is very different than we imagined. Brian was in our home most every day in May staying with Ken while I ran the bus route with kids. Mike Powell, loved deeply by Ken and unknown to me until the research treatment, has a heart being shaped to run hard after God and his protective posture of me and CJ has created space for change. The agency has been protected because of Tom's willingness to ask questions in order to learn about the HIV infected population and their needs and to "do the books". Carol Murray's passion and energy, given when she had little to give due to her family obligations, has caused the decisions to be considered and prayed about and reconsidered. Furthermore, Carol's regard for me has brought resources that help me take the next step in this journey with God that will continue to write my story that is one requiring others to risk and to hope and live faith and love enough to participate in it.

So, what is the next step? There is no blueprint but this I know God has a destiny for me that declares a need for sanctuary! God's people are the only agents that can stand arms linked to create truth, hope, faith and love. Are we very good at linking together? Do we on purpose try to create a sense of belongingness for people with HIV or AIDS? Have we learned how to be Jesus without talking much? Is it really possible that believers from various churches work together? How often do believers get out of their comfort zone? This I know, God wants His people to be kindness, love, patience, provision of need and hope to hurting people. And I know people living or affected by HIV/AIDS hurt.

This is an odd comment, but it has been part of my journey since June 2nd, 2002. Ken's vision was not a big place full of HIV infected/ affected people. It was not expanding in five different locations and it was not about a monument to his life. The vision in Ken's heart that birthed Casa Gloriosa was that God's people become sturdy, that they risk comfort and convenience, that they try and fail and try again and that they give up their dirt to God's Spirit who can and will make them useful. He believed that HIV/AIDS was a tool, the tool Ken had, to spur the people of faith to a point of discontent. If a believer is with a discontented heart where can he go but into the presence of God? And in God's presence there is hope, energy, unity and power. Power to find creative ways to lift the name that name above all names, Jesus, high without saying one word!

The agency of Casa Gloriosa has done the work assigned for it. The vision does not end, the entity may be modified but the work that was provided cannot be maintained because the system of care, Ken & Johna, is no more. That has been difficult for me to accept. I will briefly tell you the process by which I've come to this point.

Ken died, we had the memorials, and I got as busy as I could with work to maintain the status quo of Casa Gloriosa. John Aker, in a meeting about something, asked how I was doing and I fell apart. I shared with him that I lacked willingness and that really I could not claim a willing to be willing status. He shared with me from the book of Mark about the leper that asked Jesus to heal him saying "you can if you will." And Jesus said, "I will." Pastor John's words were much more precise and eloquent than I can state but from our exchange I realized that it was necessary for me to learn that when I can't He will and even when I have no will for the call of God He will. My query to God became how? How God can I experience you?

God is good! I need and want, no, want isn't a strong enough word; I desire and yearn for an experience in God's presence. There are gifts in me, God's anointing is on me and I have skill but none of that is enough for me without a new exchange with God. His presence, a face-to-face exchange, is what I must have. And again the question is how? I don't know so I wait. That sounds simple until I tried to wait. My process required that I became still [no more Johna generated noise] so I could listen to His word for me [not my want or opinion or the directive of any other] and in that place of stillness and quietness I can wait.

The Board of Directors will take the agency through the paces for transition that is respectful to clients, donors and to me and to God. God will use me, and CJ, in the community of people who are HIV infected and affected to exhort, to call, to challenge and to partner with believers willing to risk enough to be part of this continuing story that is to the glory of God. And until I know that I know that I know, I wait.

www.ingramcontent.com/pod-product-compliance
Lightning Source LLC
Chambersburg PA
CBHW061312280526
45784CB00002B/966

* 9 7 8 1 4 3 4 3 2 3 7 6 7 *